...sed HIV/AIDS care

Home-based HIV/AIDS care

Leana Uys; Sue Cameron (Eds)

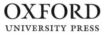

OXFORD
UNIVERSITY PRESS

OXFORD

UNIVERSITY PRESS

Great Clarendon Street, Oxford OX2 6DP

Oxford University Press is a department of the University of Oxford.
It furthers the University's objective of excellence in research, scholarship,
and education by publishing worldwide in

Oxford New York

Auckland Bangkok Buenos Aires Cape Town Chennai
Dar es Salaam Delhi Hong Kong Istanbul Karachi Kolkata
Kuala Lumpur Madrid Melbourne Mexico City Mumbai Nairobi
São Paulo Shanghai Taipei Tokyo Toronto

with an associated company in Berlin

Oxford is a registered trade mark of Oxford University Press
in the UK and in certain other countries

Published in South Africa
by Oxford University Press Southern Africa, Cape Town

Home-based HIV/AIDS care

ISBN 0 19 578198 8

© Oxford University Press Southern Africa 2003

Commissioning editor: Arthur Attwell
Editor: Emily Bowles
Designer and cover designer: Mark Standley
Photographer: Louise Gubb
Cover photograph: Louise Gubb
Medical proofreader: Dr Bridget Farham
Indexer: Jeanne Cope

Published by Oxford University Press Southern Africa
PO Box 12119, N1 City, 7463, Cape Town, South Africa

Set in 10,5 pt on 13,35 pt Minion by RHT desktop publishing, Durbanville
Reproduction by RHT desktop publishing
Cover reproduction by The Image Bureau
Printed and bound by ABC Press, Epping, Cape Town

Please note: People photographed for this publication are not
necessarily living with HIV/AIDS.

Contents

Contributors

Stefan Blom MA Clinical Psychology (Stellenbosch), is a clinical psychologist and consultant from Cape Town. He is the director of the Counselling and Psychological Empowerment Consultancy (CAPE), and is a practising family therapist.

Carey Bremridge MA Clinical Psychology (Stellenbosch), is currently the manager of the HIV/AIDS programme of the University of Stellenbosch. She previously worked at Stellenbosch AIDS Action, a non-profit organization providing training, counselling, testing, and support to HIV-infected and -affected people. In addition, she works as an HIV/AIDS trainer, training peer/lay counsellors in the private and public health sectors. She is a part-time lecturer in community psychology and runs a small private practice.

Sue Cameron BA (Hons) Unisa, is Head of the Education and Training Department at Pretoria Sungardens Hospice and has been involved in the field of HIV/AIDS since 1988. She develops training material related to different aspects of HIV/AIDS, runs workshops, and works with patients and their families.

Kath Defilippi registered nurse and midwife, worked as a midwifery tutor prior to starting the South Coast Hospice home-care programme in 1983. She introduced rural outreach in 1986, which laid the foundation for the integrated community-based home care-model that was implemented in the area at the beginning of 1997. She is currently CEO of South Coast Hospice and convenor of the Hospice Association of South Africa's patient care and education sub-committee.

Liz Gwyther MB Ch.B. and MFGP Diploma in Palliative Medicine (Cardiff), is convenor for the postgraduate programmes in palliative medicine at the

University of Cape Town. She has been involved in hospice care on a voluntary basis since 1995. She has been active in training and development for community-based home care for HIV/AIDS care with hospices in the Western Cape. She was also involved in the development of the first in-patient palliative care unit in Cape Town. She is CEO of St Luke's Hospice, Chairperson of the Hospice Association of the Western Cape, a member of the education sub-committee of the Hospice Association of South Africa (HASA), and a member of the HASA board.

Jill Knott BA Social Work (Hons) (Wits), worked as a probation officer for the Department of Social Welfare for four years. She then worked for the Johannesburg City Council, working for three years with tuberculosis patients and supervising the work of social workers in Soweto. Employed by Wits Hospice since 1987, she has worked as intake officer, and full-time social worker. She is at present Head of the Psycho-social Service Department at Wits and of Soweto Hospices, as well as responsible for the Centre for Palliative Learning at Hospice Wits. Her experience with HIV/AIDS has been in counselling patients, their partners, and their families and doing bereavement counselling for people who have experienced the death of someone from HIV/AIDS. She has also been involved in training volunteers and various members of the community in HIV/AIDS awareness.

Joan Marston B.Soc.Sc. (Nursing), is Executive Director of Naledi Hospice and The St Nicholas Children's Hospice in the Free State. She is also Advocacy Officer for the Hospice Association of South Africa and has been involved with palliative care, home-based care, and training for twelve years. She has a special interest in the care of children and bereavement counselling.

Rose Smart BA (Psychology) and Nursing, has worked in the field of HIV/AIDS since 1991, first with the Pietermaritzburg Chamber of Commerce and Industries, then as Manager of the Pietermaritzburg AIDS Training, Information and Counselling Centre (ATICC). She joined the National Aids Programme as a consultant and then as director until 1999. In 2000, she was commissioned by the National AIDS and Children Task Team (NACTT) to conduct a rapid appraisal of children living with HIV/AIDS in South Africa, and subsequently acted as the managing consultant for Save the Children when they commissioned a range of studies to inform the debate around affected children. Since then she has been a consultant focusing on HIV/AIDS-affected children, community-based HIV/AIDS initiatives such as home-based care, and developing workplace and multisectoral responses.

Leana Uys D.Soc.Sc. (Nursing), is currently Professor of Nursing and Director of the WHO Collaborating Centre for Nursing and Midwifery at the University of Natal. She has been involved in HIV/AIDS research, and as external moderator in the national palliative care course offered by the South African Hospice Association.

Laura Ziady B.Soc.S. (Nursing), Diplomas in Nursing Admin and Education, Certificates in Palliative Nursing Science and Infection Control Nursing, is the unit manager of the Infection Control Department of Bloemfontein Medi-Clinic; a part time lecturer at the Free State University School of Nursing; and a part-time caregiver and educator for Naledi Hospice (Bloemfontein), and Bloemfontein AIDS Training, Information and Counselling Centre (ATICC). She has been involved with HIV/AIDS training, patient care, and health care, and with staff training regarding HIV/AIDS since 1989.

List of abbreviations

AIDS	Acquired Immune Deficiency Syndrome
ARC	AIDS-related complex
ART	antiretroviral therapy
CBO	community-based organization
CCG	community caregiver
CINDI	children in distress
DOTS	directly-observed treatment short course
FBO	faith-based organization
FCG	family or friend caregiver
HIV	Human Immunodeficiency Virus
ICBHC	Integrated Community-Based Home Care
NGO	non-governmental organization
PCG	primary caregiver, usually a family member
PLHA	person or people living with HIV/AIDS
TB	tuberculosis
VCT	voluntary counselling and testing for HIV

Acknowledgement

The editors wish to thank all the authors who worked together so willingly on this project. We also wish to thank the photographer, Louise Gubb, who donated her time and talent to this project in support of home-care in this country.

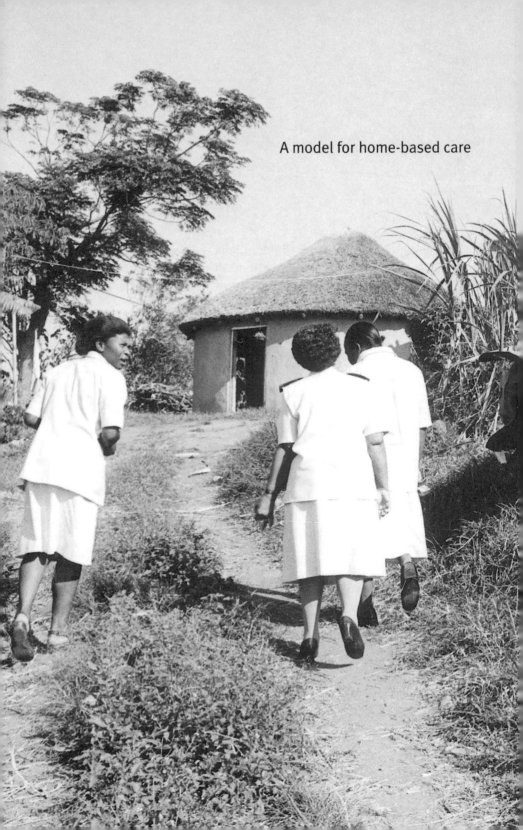

A model for home-based care

1 | A model for home-based care

Leana Uys

Introduction

As early as 1986, the Committee on a National Strategy for AIDS (CNSA) for the USA described the system of AIDS care in terms of three components, namely hospital care, out-patient care, and community-based care. They described the main functions of each component as follows:

- *Hospitals:* Diagnosis and in-patient therapy, and discharge planning to integrate patients with out-patient and community agencies.
- *Out-patient services:* Medical management of patients with AIDS-related complex (ARC) or acquired immune deficiency syndrome (AIDS), ideally delivered through dedicated AIDS clinics, as well as counselling and health education.
- *Community-based care:* This is care occurring at a patient's residence to supplement or replace hospital-based care. This includes medication management (including infusions), palliative care, and social support (CNSA 1986).

Home-care programmes started in North America and Europe when it became clear that hospital care was too expensive, and that families and other carers found it difficult to cope on their own with the demanding care of people living with HIV/AIDS (PLHA) (Spier and Edwards 1990). In the USA, CNSA concluded that:

> If the care of these patients is to be both comprehensive and cost-effective, it must be conducted as much as possible in the community, with hospitalization only when necessary. The various requirements for the care of patients with asymptomatic HIV infection, AIDS-Related Complex, or AIDS (i.e. community-based care, outpatient care, hospitalization) should be carefully coordinated (CNSA 1986, 19).

There are now well-developed home-care systems in most African countries, although coverage and access is still not universal. Home-based care is usually given by a family or friend caregiver (FCG), supported by a trained community caregiver (CCG).

Home-based care entails the provision of needed health care by a primary caregiver to a patient or family at home, often supported by a CCG. A primary caregiver (PCG) is an informal caregiver that may be the biological mother or father, a grandparent, friend, or foster or adoptive parent who provides most of the care to the PLHA at home (Zimba and McInerney 2001). A CCG is a community member who is trained to assist the PCG through direct care and support.

The focus of home-based care is:

- the PLHA
- the FCG, and
- the children of the household.

The person living with HIV/AIDS

From the moment the diagnosis is made, the PLHA needs counselling and teaching. Later on the person needs nursing care. During the whole process of the illness they will need emotional and spiritual support, and often also economic support. In a recent study conducted in South Africa it was found that patients seen by CCGs can fall anywhere on the ill-healthy continuum. (See Table 1.1)

Table 1.1 Condition of patients seen by community caregivers

Patient condition	% of total
Patient is without major symptoms	16%
Patient has been very ill, but is now better	28%
Patient is acutely ill with an infection	9%
Patient is very weak, but can still get out of bed	29%
Patient is bedridden	19%

Source: Uys 2002

The family or friends caring for the person

This group needs much counselling and teaching to be able to cope emotionally and physically with the illness of the loved one. The involvement with the family may commence at disclosure, and end after the death of the patient.

The children in the household

Children might be orphaned or otherwise affected by the illness of parents or siblings. It has become increasingly clear that home-based care programmes are one of the most suitable avenues for launching orphan care in a community.

Benefits of home-based care

The benefits of home-based care are as follows:
- It allows the patient and the family time to come to grips with the illness, and the impending death of the patient.
- It is less expensive for the family because problems such as transport to hospital, time spent on hospital visits, and other costs are reduced. Relatives can take care of the patient while attending to other chores.
- Care is more personalized, and the PLHA feels less isolated from family and friends.
- People prefer to face ill health and death in familiar surroundings rather than in a hospital ward.
- The totality of care is less expensive for the country than institutional options, since periods of hospitalization are reduced (Uys 2001a).

Models for home-based care

Over the years, a number of different systems have been developed to offer home-based care, namely:
- integrated home-based care
- single service home-based care, and
- informal home-based care.

Integrated home-based care

The integrated home-based care model works by linking all the service providers with patients and their families in a continuum of care. It endeavours to enhance mutual support and collaboration between different components (families, CCGs, clinics, hospitals, support groups, non-governmental organizations [NGOs], and community-based organizations [CBOs]). This system allows for referral between all partners as trust is built, and it develops capacity in all partners. It ensures that CCGs are trained, and then supervised and supported. Figure 1.1 depicts one model of this kind of care. It illustrates the central position of the PLHA, the family, and the small network around the patient. This small group is supported by a large and growing network of services, and should also be supported by the larger community. All the care is given based on palliative care standards, and is ultimately aimed at preventing the illness by increasing openness and understanding, and thereby changing behaviour (Louden 1999).

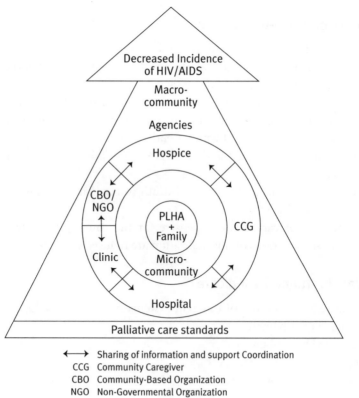

Figure 1.1 The integrated home-based care model

Source: Uys 2001b

Single service home-based care

In the single service home-based care setting, one service component (a hospital, a clinic, a NGO, or a church) organizes home-based care by recruiting volunteers, training them, and linking them with patients and their families at home.

Informal home-based care

In the informal home-based care setting, families care for their members at home, with the informal assistance of their own social network. Nobody has any specific training or external support, and there is no organization.

It would be ideal if all home-based care could be delivered through an integrated model. This approach ensures that the patient and family get all the help they need, from the day the diagnosis is made, through all the phases to terminal care. The family even gets support after the death of the patient. It also ensures that the quality of care is optimal, since there is supervision and support for the CCGs, and different services assist each other in improving care.

However, one often has to start by taking the individual service approach until other partners can be recruited and involved. Informal care is very taxing, since the FCG may lack the necessary skill, knowledge, and emotional support.

Care given

Counselling and teaching

The tasks most often performed by CCGs are counselling and giving information (94 per cent of visits), and giving psychological and emotional support (45 per cent of visits) (Uys 2001a). Therefore, counselling and teaching are among the most important skills a CCG has to have.

The objectives of the counselling and teaching task are to:
- promote a positive acceptance of the diagnosis
- promote disclosure, especially to sexual partners and FCGs
- enhance understanding of the illness and a healthy lifestyle
- assist with preparation for death, such as child care, and
- assist the family to deal with loss.

The counselling includes pre-test and post-test counselling, helping the PLHA and their family to live with the diagnosis, dealing with disclosure, preparing for death, and providing bereavement counselling to families. It is a highly valued part of the CCG's work. In cases where there are children in the household, the role could also involve giving special attention and support to child-headed households, and child care and respite facilities for carers.

Palliative care

According to the International Hospice Institute and College (IHIC) 'Palliative care is comprehensive care of people with active progressive far advanced disease for whom the prognosis is limited and the focus of care is the quality of life' (Doyle, et al. 1993, 26). CCGs assist FCGs and patients with aspects such as hygiene (28 per cent of visits), wound care (13 per cent of visits) and symptom control (68 per cent of visits) (Uys 2002). The objectives of this task are to improve the quality of life of the patient and family by:

- making the patient more comfortable
- improving the health of the patient, and
- lightening the care load on the FCG.

Symptom control demands specialist input. In this regard specialist organizations such as the Hospice Association could make an important contribution.

In terms of terminal care, five elements make up a 'good death' (Mak and Clinton 1999, 56–65). These include comfort, openness, completion, control, optimism, readiness, and choice of location. Much has been written about how to achieve these elements in assisting PLHA, and each one poses an enormous challenge.

Organization of a home-care service

The essential components of setting up a home-based care system are:

- establishing a dedicated management team
- managing CCGs
- setting up a system
- finding resources
- establishing support groups, and
- doing research.

A dedicated management team

In a national evaluation of such programmes (Uys 2001a), the need for a skilled management team with a vision for home-based care was seen as a priority for success. It is a great help if the team can get people from different services involved in the continuum of care.

Management of community caregivers

CCGs have to be recruited, trained, supervised, and supported. CCGs are usually recruited from the communities in which they will work. Because of the complexity of the counselling and physical needs of clients, a training period of at least three weeks is recommended. After training, they should be allocated to a specific area, and a professional should supervise their work, if at all possible. This will not only promote quality of care, but will also act as a support for the CCG. This is an emotionally and physically demanding job, and support of the CCG is essential.

Setting up a system

A home-based care system includes the following:
- *Recruitment:* There should be clear ways for clients, and people who want to refer clients, to contact the service. The service must be known to the community, and access by telephone and/or a physical address should be established.
- *Policies:* The management should establish policies for the functioning of the service to prevent problems as far as possible. The following policies might be necessary:
  - job description for CCGs
  - conditions of service of CCGs
  - financial policy
  - policy on confidentiality and disclosure
  - care policies, for example guidelines for dealing with specific symptoms, and
  - referrals policy between different service components.
- *Procedures:* Home-based care services follow different procedures. In some settings CCGs go to the nearest clinic, where they get the names and addresses of clients from the nurse. In other settings, they go from house to house looking for any sick person who needs assistance, and in this way

they trace PLHA. In some settings they walk from client to client, and in others they use public transport or a dedicated vehicle. The system of work needs to be developed depending on the situation. CCGs need assistance with deciding how often to visit different clients, and how to prioritize their work in the face of overwhelming demands. Procedures need to be established to deal with these issues.

- *Recording:* Decisions have to be made about the level of record-keeping by CCGs. Simple statistical recording of each visit, each new contact, potential orphans, and each admission of death is essential for future planning, for funding proposals, and for accountability. Depending on the skills of the CCGs, it might be possible to keep more sophisticated records of the condition of the clients.

Finding resources

No service can run without resources. The management will have to access resources to support the care given by CCGs. In many projects the CCGs are paid a minimum salary, or are at least provided with money for transport. Equipment such as bedpans, linen protectors, gloves, and towels might also be needed.

PLHAs and their families often live in poverty (Sliep, et al. 2001). It is almost impossible to be involved in home-based care without getting involved in poverty relief. Food parcels, clothes, assistance with school fees, and other urgent economic needs make it essential that the home-care service links up with a social welfare service to deal with this aspect.

Resources also include human and service resources. The management should ensure that CCGs have access to a social worker, a skilled counsellor, legal assistance, and consultants for medical issues. Without such a network, the home-based care could be of a poor quality, leading to disenchantment of patients and their families. The key word here is 'network', since it would be impossible to employ all these specialists. The management team should link with existing individuals and agencies and use the resources in their service.

Support groups

Community-based support groups are an economical way of reaching PLHA and their PCGs. Such groups usually meet once a week in an accessible location. The time is used for counselling and teaching, for socializing and support, and for income generation and handing out of food parcels or other assistance that is available. It can also be used for directly observed treatment short-course (DOTS) surveillance and the handing out of medication.

A good example of the use of these groups is found in the Zululand Hospice home-based care programme. Here, support groups meet at four different settings to enable clients to get to the meetings more easily. The meetings take place once a week at each setting. The buildings are very basic; one is a nursery school that is used from 12h00 only. Another is an empty room in the homestead of a CCG. For each PLHA one FCG is allowed to attend, but there are often more family members. While the group is busy with educational talks, prayers, handwork or singing, the CCG and the supervising registered nurse (RN) see individuals for counselling and assessment. Each person is also given bread, peanut butter, jam, and a cooldrink.

Research

Having access to the home and family provides caregivers with the opportunity to obtain valuable information that can impact on local, provincial, and even national planning. For example, research could show:

- what factors need to be in place in order for impoverished PLHA to comply with tuberculosis (TB) treatment
- what support measures enable families to cope with caring for a person with full-blown AIDS at home
- how nutrition improves with education and referral to community gardens
- what impact a home-care programme has on the micro-community in terms of their acceptance and support of PLHA and their families
- how partnerships with traditional healers can be established
- what motivation the community needs in order to respond to the needs of its vulnerable children
- how the care given by paid caregivers compares with that given by volunteers
- what it takes to have a network of volunteers supporting a core of paid CCGs, and
- how the home-care programme impacts on hospital bed occupancy.

Project organizers should try to get academic or other research partners involved, who can take on the research responsibility. The results of research can be used to shape the future development of the project, and to assist with communication about the project and its results.

Issues in home-based care

Volunteers

The valid concern regarding the ongoing sustainability of programmes prior-itizes the use of volunteers as a cost-saving measure. When these volunteers are themselves impoverished, this poses both an ethical and economic dilemma. They too have human rights and should not be exploited. Because of their poor income and lack of opportunity, such 'volunteers' often hope that volun-teering will lead to remuneration that will enable them to improve their own and their families' lots. Exploiting their vulnerability is not to be commended.

A great deal of training is invested in home-care volunteers. This gives them additional skills and confidence and, in some instances, makes them employ-able. It is only right and natural that such people grasp any opportunity for paid employment that comes their way. This is likely to happen repeatedly. Having to train new people can be as costly to the organization as paying a nominal salary would have been.

From the quality of care perspective, there is great value in maintaining the type of continuity that is the product of a settled group of caregivers. A good home-care programme will decrease the need for hospitalization, which is a major cost saving.

Having said all that, it is also true that there are many people who are able and willing to work as volunteers. It is also true that many projects will never get off the ground without such people. Project managers and the community at large should weigh up all these factors when planning home-based care projects.

The case for professional supervision

The number of laypeople accepted for training should depend on the avail-ability of professional supervisors. PLHA requiring home-based care are criti-cally ill and need skilled physical treatment and care over and above the psycho-social support and acceptance that means so much to them and their families. People this ill would under normal circumstances be hospitalized and given round-the-clock professional care. In the light of the devastating HIV/AIDS pandemic currently raging in sub-Saharan Africa, this is not feasi-ble because of sheer numbers. Hospitals cannot cope and are in danger of being overwhelmed (Uys 2001b). PLHA therefore have the right to expect that the home care they receive is quality care, and that it forms part of a comprehensive package. This is one reason why the Integrated Community-Based Home Care (ICBHC) model developed by the Hospice Association of South Africa insists on professional supervision. The other reason indirectly benefits PLHA, in that its main objective is to mentor and nurture caregivers so as to prevent burnout and renew and replenish them emotionally and spiritually. They, in turn, are then able to empower and support the primary caregivers in the home and maintain their sense of vocation.

Appropriately, the selection criteria for professional supervisors are dealt with in the chapter on training (Chapter 3). Job descriptions need to be adjusted to incorporate the supervision of CCGs, and time has to be scheduled for the selected professionals to be trained as supervisors. The duration of training will vary according to specific disciplines and individual backgrounds and experience.

Ethics of home-based care

There are many ethical dilemmas around caring for people with HIV/AIDS. The ethical principles are as follows:

- A patient has the right to confidentiality about the diagnosis. This means that health care providers should not disclose the HIV-positive status of the patient, or the diagnosis, to others without the expressed permission of the patient.
- In cases where a patient is a danger to others, the health care provider has a duty to prevent such danger, even if it means breaking the confidentiality rule. In many cases the sexual partner(s) of a patient does not know that the person is HIV-positive, thus endangering them. Similarly, caregivers are often not informed of the patient's HIV status.

These two principles may oppose each other in a given situation, thus posing an ethical dilemma. The best policy is to promote disclosure by the patient for those people who need to know, and to support the patient if the disclosure is difficult to manage emotionally.

It is also important that managers of home-care projects protect their clients from unplanned identification. If a service is known only to care for HIV/AIDS patients, the presence of the workers from that service alone identifies the household as having an HIV-positive member. It is, therefore, usually better to work with all seriously ill people needing home care, rather than to restrict the clients to those with HIV/AIDS.

Home-care projects might from time to time take visitors on home visits, often for purposes of raising funds for the work. This might include members of the media. In order to promote the safety of the clients, media should be screened, and only those willing to accept the requirements laid down by the clients and the service providers should be allowed access to patients and their families. A media policy from one home care agency is attached in Appendix A as an example.

Ethical issues should also be dealt with in the training and supervision of community caregivers and volunteers. Ethical conduct should be frequently reinforced in discussions and carefully observed in all cases.

Conclusion

There are currently still thousands of PLHA and their families who are not being cared for by a dedicated home-based care team. Where such programmes have been implemented and evaluated, PLHA and their carers, as well as health service providers are all convinced of their intrinsic value (Uys 2001b). Therefore, a need exists for more such services to be set up. This is not one agency's task, but the responsibility of every community in the country. Even without experience, one can begin to work through the process of establishing such a service, and get appropriate advice and assistance from those with experience.

References

CNSA (Committee on a National Strategy for AIDS). 1986. *Confronting AIDS: Directions for Public Health, Health Care and Research.* Washington: National Academy Press.

Doyle, D., Hanks, G.W., and N. MacDonald. 1993. *Oxford Textbook of Palliative Medicine.* Oxford: Oxford University Press.

Louden, M. 1999. *South Coast Hospice's Community-Based HIV/AIDS Home Care Model.* HIV/AIDS Best Practice Series. Pretoria: Department of Health.

Mak, J.M.H., and M. Clinton. 1999. 'Promoting a good death: An agenda for outcomes research – a review of the literature'. *Nursing Ethics* 6 (2): 97–106.

Sliep, Y., Poggenpoel M., and A. Gmeiner. 2001. 'The experience of HIV reactive patients in rural Malawi'. *Curationis* 24 (3): 56–65.

Spier, A. and E. Edwards. 1990. *Facing AIDS: A Strategy Manual.* McGregor: SYNCOM Publishing.

Uys, L. R. 2001a. 'Evaluation of the Integrated Community-Based Home Care model'. *Curationis* 24 (3): 75–82.

Uys, L. R. 2001b. 'The implementation of the integrated community-based home care model for people living with AIDS'. *Africa Journal of Nursing and Midwifery* 3 (1): 34–41.

Uys, L.R. 2002. 'The practice of community caregivers in a home-based HIV/AIDS project in South Africa'. *Journal of Clinical Nursing* 11: 99–108.

Zimba, E.W. and P.A. McInerney. 2001. 'The knowledge and practices of primary caregivers regarding home-based care of HIV/AIDS children in Blantyre (Malawi)'. *Curationis* 24 (3): 75–90.

Implementing integrated community-based home care

2 Implementing integrated community-based home care

Kath Defilippi

Introduction

This chapter aims to deal with all the issues around setting up a home-based care programme in a specific community. The Integrated Community-based Home Care (ICHC) model described briefly in Chapter 1 is used as the framework for this chapter. This means that we follow an inclusive approach, incorporating all care providers, and not just working with the home-based care end of the continuum of care.

Preparation

The initial vision for a home-based care programme could come from people within any one of the health care providers or from somebody wishing to establish a community-based organization (CBO). In terms of the ICHC model, the idea would, at the outset, need to be shared with the other partner institutions and key figures from the community. It would also be wise to get at least one representative of people living with HIV/AIDS (PLHA) on board as a consultant from the very beginning of the planning phase (Tarantola and van Praag 2001).

Community needs assessment

Numerous groups and organizations need to be consulted in order to get an accurate picture of the community. The local council should have an HIV/ AIDS plan in place that documents HIV/AIDS needs and resources in the health district. Once a relationship has been established with hospital and primary health care clinic staff, they can be asked what impact the HIV/AIDS pandemic has had on their institutions, and what happens to PLHA who are discharged.

This is a good indicator regarding the need for home-based care. Existing organizations for PLHA will have valuable information with regard to available services. Churches may have groups involved, or prepared to become involved, in providing care and support for PLHA. If there is a hospice in the area they will definitely already be giving home-based care and will be a valuable resource that may be prepared to offer mentorship and support to a new home-based care programme. There could also be a coordinating body with whom to liaise. The Network Action Group (NAG) in the most southern Health District of KwaZulu-Natal is one such body that functions very effectively.

Funding

While community ownership goes some way towards sustaining a programme, there is no such thing as a sustainable 'free' service, even if everybody involved starts off as a volunteer. It is, therefore, ideal to source funding before starting a service and raising community expectations. Table 2.1 sets out the approximate costs of the ICHC model.

A transparent proposal that outlines who, what, where, how, when, and, most importantly, why the proposed home-based care programme is a good idea, needs to be submitted to potential donors. Clearly defined projects are easier for donor organizations to support than a poorly defined one that seems disorganized. When defining your project, be as specific as possible in describing your goals and how you intend reaching them.

Many national corporations have an allocated budget for community needs. It is not clever to apply blindly for funding. Make enquiries and find out exactly what criteria apply and what amounts are usually given, before writing a proposal. Some companies have their own application form as well as set dates for considering requests for funding. Establishing a relationship with the relevant person in the donor organization is a good investment of time and energy. This is usually done telephonically.

Ask networking partners to give constructive criticism on your draft proposal and be open to making amendments. Allow sufficient time (at least two weeks), and ensure that there are no mistakes in the final typed application. It also needs to include a clear budget. It is important to create a good first impression. Potential donors are more likely to 'help those who help themselves', so include any relevant fundraising or cost sharing plans as well as in kind contributions from the local community.

Table 2.1 Cost of an integrated community-based home-care programme

Item (in 2000)	Cost in rands	Notes
Setting up costs:		
• Training cost	R7 145	For 3 weeks of training only for 2 CCGs
• Equipment	R10 379	A very basic list of home-care equipment
• Planning	R12 146	Meetings to set up an integrated programme
Total per site	R29 670	
Running costs for one year:		
• For a site with a vehicle	R50 600	2 CCGs looking after 30 clients at any time
• For a site without a vehicle	R28 400	The same

Source: Uys and Hensher 2002, 625

The Government also needs to be approached for funding, notably the local, provincial, and national Departments of Health and Social Development (Welfare).

It is wise to use local resources first, even though support from outside of the community may be required. If only part of the funds come from external sources, it will be easier for the project to survive if these funds are cut off (Granich and Mermin 1999).

Community ownership

Ideally, every sector of the community should be able to identify with the programme of care. This ownership goes a long way towards ensuring the continuity of the service. Motivated communities validate and support home care volunteers. In addition to mobilizing local resources, the demonstration of meaningful community involvement positively impacts on the likelihood of acquiring outside funds.

Therefore, it makes sense to identify a broad spectrum of community leaders and invite them to participate during the planning and design phase of the project. If the objective is to make sure that the programme is not perceived to be party political, denominational, or in any way exclusive, discretion and careful selection of key community figures is required. Including PLHA and traditional healers also increases the likelihood of acceptance of any new programme, in that they are more inclined to endorse something that they feel part of. Community members are likely to be impressed by honesty and transparency, and will be on the lookout for any signs of empire building.

Considerable time needs to be scheduled for meetings. A balance of flexibility and firmness should characterize negotiations. Every point of view deserves to be given full attention, but once decisions have been made they need to be adhered to. An overriding consideration of all concerned has to be the attainment of the best possible quality of life for PLHA and their families, while empowering them to cope with the demands of care, grief, and loss.

The more control people from the community have of the project, the more they think of it as their own. Accountability to the community remains important throughout all the phases of programme development. A board of directors drawn from the local community governs most successful non-governmental organizations (NGOs).

Networking partners

To identify the existing community resources, ask many people, with differing backgrounds, about their experience in this regard, and follow up every lead.

One needs to have an unambiguous mission statement and be clear about the criteria of admission to the home-based care programme before making an appointment for discussions with any potential networking partners.

Together with ongoing communication, honesty with regard to limitations and a willingness to share expertise and resources make for successful networking. It is liberating to adopt a mindset of collaboration in place of competition. When organizations work together unselfishly for the ultimate good of the community they invariably benefit individually as well as collectively. Working together is greatly enhanced when a directory of community resources and a referral system is available to all the role players.

The magnitude of the HIV/AIDS pandemic makes cooperation imperative (Campbell 2001). This fact is recognized by donor organizations in that they often request a list of networking partners when processing funding applications.

Selection and training of community caregivers

It makes sense to have decided on a job description for community caregivers (CCGs) before people are selected for training. For a sample job description refer to Appendix B. The date, venue, and maximum number of candidates should also have been determined.

In addition to appropriate experience and emotional maturity, a history of community involvement, a respectful attitude, generosity of spirit, keenness to learn, and the ability to communicate effectively are valuable attributes for potential caregivers. Awareness about HIV/AIDS and a positive attitude towards PLHA is also significant, as is the perceived potential for working in a team and under professional supervision.

The ability to relate well to people is usually accompanied by a balanced lifestyle, a positive outlook, and a sense of humour.

Prospective trainees should be interviewed by a panel, which should include PLHA and community representation. Panel members need to agree on the criteria that will be applied prior to the interviews. Many of these can be incorporated into application forms. By eliminating unsuitable candidates this practice prevents both parties from wasting time and transport costs.

Some of the people who apply for training will be hoping that this will lead to a job. Transparency and upfront communication regarding the volunteer status and/or criteria for selection for a paid position, as well as the number of any potential jobs is, therefore, necessary and should preferably be backed up in writing.

Please refer to Chapter 3: *Training community caregivers for a home-based care programme,* for more information on this important topic.

Planning for sustainability

In these difficult times it is not possible to have a cast-iron guarantee of sustainability. Involving the community and earning their respect and that of health care professionals and donor organizations is probably the best way of ensuring the continuity of a home-based care programme.

One way of doing this is to incorporate a policy of monitoring and evaluation that is linked to ongoing training. Both the clinical and administrative aspects of the programme need to be vigilantly assessed on an ongoing basis. Scrupulous financial management and control, accurate statistics, and punctuality regarding the submission of reports are as important as having a reputation for giving quality care.

The scale of the HIV/AIDS pandemic and its impact in terms of the tragedy of unparalleled human loss and suffering, as well as the associated economic calamity, has made it compulsory to focus on prevention. Consequently, there is a moral and ethical obligation to link care to prevention at every possible opportunity. It is also probable that programmes with this focus will be favourably considered for funding in an environment that is bound to become more financially constrained (Health Development Networks 2001).

Providing home-based care

Meeting the following needs forms the basis of a comprehensive package of care. The needs and resources of the relevant community, formal health care system, and networking NGOs and/or faith-based organizations (FBOs) will determine the specifics in terms of how these essential needs are met:

- *Clinical management:* Providing early diagnosis, including HIV testing, appropriate prophylaxis, treatment of opportunistic infections, and effective management of pain and symptom control.
- *Nursing care:* Promoting and maintaining hygiene and nutrition; teaching the family and micro-community basic nursing skills as well as emergency measures; supervising the taking of medication and directly observed treatment short-course (DOTS) for tuberculosis (TB); teaching and facilitating the observance of universal precautions.
- *Psycho-spiritual support:* Providing counselling and spiritual support, including stress and risk reduction planning, promoting and supporting the acceptance and disclosure of serostatus; enabling coping in terms of positive living; and planning for the future of the family (in particular the placement of children).
- *Social support:* Providing welfare services and legal advice; providing information and referrals between the partners who make up the care network, including poverty alleviation and pastoral and bereavement care; facilitating peer support (Tarantola and van Praag 2001 and Ferris, et al. 1995).

The delivery of care in one particular setting

The process of care described here occurs in the southernmost Health District of KwaZulu-Natal. It is an example of a comprehensive package of holistic care that is available to PLHA along a continuum that extends from pre-diagnosis to bereavement follow-up. The ICHC model was developed in this area in 1996 as a natural progression of an established rural outreach programme.

Pre-test and post-test HIV counselling was initially provided by CCGs. This function has now been taken over by trained lay counsellors because of the high number of PLHA requiring home-based care. The availability of hospice-trained lay counsellors and rapid tests at primary health care clinics has dramatically impacted on the number of people coming forward for voluntary counselling and testing (VCT) (UNAIDS 2000).

Medical personnel at the government hospitals assume primary responsibility for the prevention and clinical management of opportunistic infections. Professional nurses from their satellite primary health care clinics and hospice, as well as the CCGs and volunteers, support them. The hospice interdisciplinary team provides expertise in the management and prevention of pain and other symptoms. This partnership between the formal health care sector and a NGO has empowered both parties with additional skills to the benefit of the PLHA, their families, and the entire community.

The home care programme is coordinated by the hospice. The ultimate responsibility for the provision of quality nursing care rests with the professional nurse supervisors. The bulk of hands-on care and teaching is provided by a core of full-time employed CCGs who are supported by an extensive network of volunteers. The hospice staff need to use vehicles because of the rural terrain, while volunteers reside within walking distance of patients' homes.

The hospice mobile teams visit each house-bound patient once a week. The volunteers provide interim care and are backed-up and professionally supervised by primary health care nurses, many of whom hold a qualification in palliative nursing care recognized by the South African Nursing Council.

The hospitals and primary health care clinics ensure that the necessary medications, including oral morphine, as well as necessary surgical supplies, are available for patients at home.

Impoverished households receive emergency food relief and gloves. Donated clothes, bedding, and toys are distributed according to need and availability. Basic home-care equipment like foam mattresses, bedpans, and walkers are loaned to PLHA from hospice stock. Volunteers and caregivers make referrals to poverty alleviation and child care projects run by networking partners.

When openness and trust prevail, many powerful teaching moments occur in the home care setting. CCGs and volunteers are skilled at using such experiential moments in terms of promoting awareness and prevention among

PLHA and their friends and relatives. Neighbours are encouraged to lend support to and care for infected and affected families.

The link between HIV/AIDS and TB is well documented. In some developing countries as many as 50 per cent of people are infected with TB (Uys 2000). Many home-care volunteers are also DOTS supervisors.

A professional nurse from either the hospice or the relevant primary health care clinic has the authority to arrange admission to hospital in the case of a home care crisis. Liaison with traditional healers has been beneficial in that they have shared knowledge regarding the use of indigenous plants as tried and tested remedies. Various skin ailments and thrush are routinely and successfully treated at home with readily available medicinal plants.

Hospice and government social workers, in collaboration with trained pastors, are involved in the direct provision of psycho-spiritual care. They also act as mentors to the rest of the care team who provide ongoing supportive counselling and are actively engaged in facilitating disclosure and promoting community acceptance of PLHA.

A children's team that comprises specially trained CCGs falls under the hospice psycho-social department. A memory box project facilitates the grief process in children and gives dying parents the opportunity of having their dreams for their children documented. Photographs, the child's birth certificate, a letter from the dying parent, and precious mementos are kept in this little metal box (see Chapter 5). The children decorate their boxes with drawings. This has developed into a form of 'play therapy' in that it facilitates them sharing what they are experiencing and feeling. Family consultations are held to make plans for the optimal placement of potential orphans. This is necessary because HIV/AIDS has severely eroded the traditional safety net of the extended family, and grandmothers, for instance, are often too tired to cope.

CCGs and volunteers refer PLHA and their families in need of welfare assistance to the hospice community social worker, who in turn liaises with colleagues employed in state institutions and relevant NGOs such as child welfare societies. Intervention from the coordinating body NAG has resulted in a system of fast tracking grants, a directory of community resources, and a referral system between all the networking partners. A Cluster Home Action Group (CHAG) has been formed to promote the placement of orphans with foster parents within the community.

PLHA who have publicly disclosed their status are nurtured and given logistical assistance in the setting up of peer support groups.

The process of home-based care in the southernmost Health District of KwaZulu-Natal

All PLHA who attend a hospital or primary health care clinic are given information regarding the availability of home care and criteria for admission to the programme. They are also given a brochure with contact details.

On receipt of a referral, the relevant hospice team:

• performs a comprehensive first assessment at their next visit to the specific geographic area

• completes a first assessment form (see Appendix C) and informs the primary health care clinic

• introduces volunteers whenever appropriate and available

• spends time listening to, and supporting, the PLHA and the primary caregiver (PCG) before drawing up a holistic care plan

• demonstrates procedures such as mouth and pressure care to the family

• dresses wounds and gives basic medications from the home-care kit, if indicated, and

• teaches universal precautions and gives the family sufficient gloves for a week.

It is a relief for PLHA and their families to know that, should a crisis occur during the week between hospice visits, immediate help would be forthcoming from the primary health care clinic. The hospice team makes weekly visits to the clinic and hospital on designated days, to maintain communication regarding patients on the home-care programme. PLHA are often transported home from hospital by the hospice vehicle.

A policy is in place that allows for straightforward re-admission to hospital should this become necessary. Despite this, local hospital records indicate that the average time spent in hospital has come down to 3.5 days per patient (Cele 2001). Given the appalling social circumstances and lack of infrastructure, this is remarkable. In some rural areas, people have to walk up to 4 km to fetch water, and many do not yet have electricity in their homes.

A professional nurse is telephonically available to CCGs and accompanies each team on home visits at least once a week. PLHA care records and statistics are collated on a monthly basis.

Monitoring and evaluation

Monitoring and evaluation are often only thought of once a programme is up and running. In fact, even the planning should be monitored and documented.

It is preferable to include this important aspect throughout, from the planning phase onwards. Much time, energy, and expense are saved when monitoring and evaluation are actively planned for. For instance, the trouble and expense involved in changing PLHA care records will be avoided if, from the outset, these have been designed to capture data that will show how effective the programme is. Accurate documentation is one of the greatest challenges associated with ICHC. Capacity building and training are necessary for laypeople to see the value of what can easily be perceived as just extra paperwork.

Ideally, monitoring and evaluation should be integrated and applied across the whole continuum of care. At the outset, standards that provide for 'attainable quality' in the specific setting need to be in place.

Once these standards have been agreed upon, they can be used to compile a guideline or protocol. Indicators can then be developed to assess the quality of care received by PLHA and their families as compared to the guideline.

It is also necessary to monitor what percentage of the population of PLHA, who meet the criteria to be on the home-care programme, are actually reached. In an integrated comprehensive model it is also important to measure what percentage of PLHA who tested positive were referred to the appropriate networking partner for clinical care or support.

According to Tarantola and van Praag (2001, 94), 'monitoring and evaluating HIV care and support is still new, and the development of effective monitoring tools and methodologies is in its early stages'. The Hospice Palliative Care Association of South Africa (HPCA), in conjunction with the University of Natal, has developed an audit tool to measure the quality of palliative care in terms of the ICBHC model. Figure 2.1 depicts a modified version of the section dealing with care in the home. The HPCA Patient Care and Education sub-committee have also developed clinical standards of care and are in the process of accrediting member hospices in South Africa.

'Factors such as gender and age and respect for non-discrimination and other human rights should provide a lens through which every monitoring and evaluation indicator is examined' (Tarantola and van Praag 2001, 102). These issues cut across every aspect of any health care service and are particularly vital during crisis periods, such as the diagnosis of a life-threatening illness and the onset of full-blown AIDS.

Regular external evaluation should take place in addition to this ongoing internal monitoring. Serious attention should also be paid to informal feedback from the community itself and from networking partners. Every complaint should be followed up.

A modification of the HPCA ICHC tool is used to audit the home-based care programme in the southernmost Health District of KwaZulu-Natal on a six-monthly basis, as depicted in Figure 2.1. The hospice in the area sought accreditation from HPCA, and was found to comply with the clinical standards of care. This accreditation is valid for four years.

Figure 2.1 Audit tool for a client or family interview

Site: **Date:**

Interviewee(s):

Choose a client who is bedridden or almost bedridden for this interview, but one who can speak and understand questions.

No.	Item	Yes	No
1	Were you given the opportunity to discuss your needs and problems?		
2	Did you feel that these were adequately addressed?		
3	Were you given sufficient information to enable you to understand and plan treatment and care?		
4	Was your pain controlled to your satisfaction?		
5	Were other symptoms controlled to your satisfaction?		
6	Did you receive support from other health professionals when you needed it to meet your needs?		
7	Were you referred to other health services when necessary?		
8	Have you received sufficient information and training from health care workers to enable you to cope at home? (Note: This item is addressed to the primary caregiver.)		

Figure 2.1 *continued*

No.	Item	Yes	No
9	Do you know how, where, and whom to contact if you need assistance?		
10	Do you feel that the health care workers have kept information concerning you and your condition confidential?		

N/A: Not applicable. Use this when an item does not apply to the client, and explain why you are doing this.

Not asked: Use this when you choose not to ask a specific question, for example you cannot ask item 10 if a family member who is not in the confidence of the client is present during the interview.

Caring for caregivers

It is only natural to feel sad and tired when one is constantly exposed to suffering and loss while doing one's job. Without support this can lead to burnout. When burnout occurs, people become despondent and lose their capacity to give compassionate care. There is an inclination to develop a negative self-image and to become convinced that it is not possible to make a positive difference. Poverty, stigma, and the plight of orphans and vulnerable children exacerbate the risk of burnout for HIV/AIDS caregivers in developing countries.

These caregivers have the additional burden of having to deal with multiple deaths of young people. It is, therefore, vital that 'care for the caregiver' is incorporated into the home-care programme. Fixed debriefing time needs to be scheduled with a suitably experienced and qualified professional, skilled in giving psycho-social support. It is simultaneously necessary to adopt a flexible approach so as to be able to respond to the needs of specific individual caregivers. Employed caregivers should receive this personal/emotional supervision during work hours.

Hospices have tried to integrate caring for the caregiver into their organizational culture:

- During the selection process an applicant's emotional coping skills, previous stressful life experiences, and current lifestyle are taken into account. It is a recognized fact that previous stressful life events can equip one with additional strength. However, unresolved previous losses and present stressors can leave a person vulnerable to developing burnout.

- Stress management is included in initial and ongoing training. The ability to recognize personal stress and to ask for help is encouraged and is not perceived as a weakness.
- Teamwork and communication between caregivers are actively promoted.
- Within reason, caregivers have permission to say no, and to limit their activities, in order to sustain their own health and wellbeing.
- Employed caregivers work a maximum of 40 hours per week.
- There is an adequate vacation allowance and a policy that leave is not accumulated.
- Social support is facilitated so that caregivers can participate in a network of caring and reciprocal relationships that make for a sense of belonging.
- Vigilance is important with regard to looking out for manifestations of stress, especially grief overload, avoidance of PLHA and their families, staff conflict, and repeated health problems (Ferris, et al. 1995).
- Planned, professional interventions for caregiver support are seen as being fundamental to the maintenance of a healthy, caring organizational environment (Ferris, et al. 1995).
- A clear policy for post-occupational exposure prophylaxis is in place.

A pivotal part of home care is providing support for the PCG in the home who carries the heaviest load in terms of providing continuous care under difficult circumstances. It is imperative that these informal caregivers are:
- taught universal precautions
- encouraged to seek emotional support by talking to a friend and/or 'counsellor'
- supported in seeking respite care to allow for periods of physical and emotional rest away from their care giving responsibilities, and
- informed of the need for, and encouraged to pursue, bereavement care following the death of their loved one (Ferris, et al. 1995).

Growth and development

As a programme becomes well known and accepted by the community, there is likely to be a greater and more diverse demand for care. In addition, the needs in communities with high HIV prevalence rates can be tremendous. With a band of committed and generous caregivers in place it is tempting, and occasionally necessary, to broaden the scope of home care. It can sometimes seem as if an established and trustworthy CBO is the group best equipped to meet a vast array of needs. While this may be true, serious discernment should be practised by such an organization. There is a real danger of losing focus and taking on more than can be effectively managed.

Another and often wiser way of dealing with the increasing amount of care and additional pressing needs, such as orphan care and poverty alleviation, is for the recognized organization to become a mentor to other groups within the community.

Conclusion

Increasing the administrative capacity of community groups, particularly with regard to financial management, is of primary importance. Learners from other organizations can be included in training courses and skills development workshops. It is hard to exaggerate the benefit derived from modelling respectful holistic care to newly trained caregivers. This can be achieved by scheduling compulsory clinical placement for students who have completed their initial caregiver training. The HPCA of South Africa has a number of member hospices with the capacity and will to become involved in mentorship programmes.

Along with programme maturity come the opportunity and obligation to measure the efficiency and effectiveness of the care continuum within the comprehensive community package. This is linked to the effectiveness of the referral system between networking partners. Documenting and publishing lessons learnt can be of immense benefit to both the formal and NGO health care sector. The credibility of the organization is enhanced as well as the prospect of sustainability. A significant contribution is made towards improving the quality of life of PLHA and their families. Having the potential to make a positive difference even beyond one's own area of operation by sharing lessons learnt, gives the members of an organization a real sense of achievement.

References

Campbell, L. 2001. *Interim report on HIV/AIDS/STD/TB Pilot site in UGU South Health District*. Port Shepstone: South Coast Hospice.

Cele, E.B. 2001. *Murchison Hospital Bed Occupancy Records.* Unpublished report from Murchison Hospital Retro Team. Port Shepstone: Murchison Hospital.

Ferris, F.D., Flannery J.S., McNeal H.B., Morissette M.R., Cameron R., and G. Bally. 1995. *A Comprehensive Guide for the Care of Persons with HIV Disease. Module 4: Palliative Care.* Toronto: Mount Sinai Hospital & Casey House Hospice.

Granich, R. and J. Mermin. 1999. *HIV Health and Your Community.* Stanford: Stanford University Press.

Health Development Networks. 2001. 'Findings and Recommendations', proceedings of the first *Southern African Regional Community Home Based Care Conference.* Gabarone: Botswana Government Printers.

Tarantola, D. and E. van Praag. 2001. 'Evaluating care programs for people living with HIV/AIDS'. In *Evaluating Programs for HIV/AIDS Prevention and Care in Developing Countries,* edited by T. Rehle, T. Saidel, S. Mills, and R. Magnani, pp. 93–102. Washington Family Health International.

UNAIDS. 2000. *Report on the Global HIV/AIDS Epidemic.* Geneva: WHO (World Health Organization).

Uys, L. R. 2000. *An Evaluation of the Implementation of the Integrated Community-based Home Care Model in South Africa.* Unpublished report for the Department of Health, Pretoria.

Uys, L.R. and M. Hensher. 2002. 'The cost of home-based terminal care for people with AIDS in South Africa'. *South African Medical Journal* 92 (8): 624–628.

Recommended reading

Van Praag, E. 2001. 'Home and community care for people living with HIV/AIDS in different cultural and economic settings'. Paper presented at the *5th International Conference on Home and Community Based Care,* Chiang Mai, Thailand, May.

Training community caregivers for a home-based care programme

3 | Training community caregivers for a home-based care programme

Sue Cameron

Introduction

Community caregivers are a key part of the integrated community-based home care (ICHC) model and work as part of the team providing care and support for PLHA and their families. In many areas, particularly those with limited health resources, these caregivers, who live and work in the community, are the mainstay of home-based care programmes.

It is essential that community caregivers (CCGs) receive proper training to provide a high standard of care. If caregivers are not equipped with the knowledge and skills they need, they will not be able to function as part of the health care team, and the home-based care programme will not succeed.

In South Africa, the *South African Qualifications Authority (SAQA) Act* (Act 58 of 1995) has created a new framework for education and training. There are currently no mechanisms in place for the accreditation of home-based care workers or ancillary health workers and the aim is to develop national standards, recognized and registered by SAQA so that home-based caregivers can access programmes and career paths and can gain accreditation and certification within the field of health care.

The Standards Generating Body (SGB) for Ancillary Health Care has, to date, developed the following unit standards that have been approved by SAQA for basic health promotion:

- Perform basic life support and first aid in both life-threatening and non-life threatening emergencies.
- Assess the interrelationship between the individual, the family, and the community in terms of primary health care issues.
- Assess the client's situation and assist the client and family to manage home-based health care.

- Explain preventive measures to prevent disasters.
- Assist the community members to access services in accordance with their health-related human rights.

The fourth unit standard above relates directly to the area of home-based care, and providers of home-based care training need to ensure that their programmes are in line with the unit standards and that they are accredited as training providers by the Education and Training Quality Assurance Body (ETQA), so that learners will be eligible for certificates from ETQA. Many of these mechanisms are not yet in place, and organizations that wish to provide home-care training should contact the Health and Welfare Sector Education and Training Authority (HWSETA) for details.[1]

Infrastructure of the home-based care training programme

When planning a training programme for CCGs, it is important to have a clear idea of the infrastructure of the home-based care programme that one is seeking to develop, so that training is designed to meet the specific needs and conditions of the care setting. One needs to have a clear idea of the:

- geographical area
- health care resources in the area (for example, hospitals, clinics, etc.)
- networking procedures
- identified needs of the community
- type of PLHA and families served by the programme
- composition of the health care team for the area
- available funding, and
- transport facilities.

This will ensure that when training takes place, it takes into consideration the specific conditions under which caregivers will be working and the range of resources that are available in any particular community. There is little value in starting a training programme until this infrastructure is in place.

Before seeking suitable learners, it is important to establish what you will be able to offer them on completion of their training, so that the issue of voluntary work or paid employment is made clear before training begins.

---

1 The Health and Welfare Sector Education and Training Authority (HWSETA) can be contacted at Private Bag X 15 Gardenview 2047. Tel No.: 011 622 6852. Fax 011 616 8939. E-mail: hwseta@hwseta.org.za

Before training can begin, the following components need to be in place:

Trainers

Selection criteria

To develop a team of trainers for the course, choose people who:
- are professional people (nurses, social workers, teachers) with an interest in community-based care and have a good knowledge of the community that the home-based care programme will serve
- are experienced in the teaching/training/facilitation of adult learners
- have good communication skills, and
- have a good command of the relevant language/languages of the area.

Role

The trainer's role will include:
- helping the learners to develop self-awareness as well as insight into their role as CCGs
- helping learners to gain knowledge
- showing learners the skills they will need
- helping learners to practise their skills
- providing opportunities for problem solving
- liaising with other organizations that will contribute to the training course, and
- liaising with hospital and clinic personnel.

Supervisors

Selection criteria

Supervisors should:
- be professional people with a good understanding of community-based care
- have leadership and organizational skills
- have the ability to commit the necessary time to the caregivers (approximately one hour per caregiver every two weeks)
- have experience and an interest in facilitation, mentoring, and counselling, and
- have access to psycho-social support for themselves.

Role

The supervisor's role will be to:
- nurture and mentor the caregivers, and
- identify and address problem areas.

Site

An accessible site that is able to provide the resources needed to run a training course needs to be identified. These resources would include:
- sufficient tables and chairs for the learners
- adequate space for group work
- adequate toilet facilities
- facilities for providing refreshments
- blackboard or whiteboard
- overhead projector and other teaching equipment
- stationery for learners, and
- equipment for practical demonstrations.

Liaison with clinic and hospital

Written arrangements need to be made with the clinic, hospital, and other training resources where the learners will spend time during their training. It is important that these arrangements are finalized before the training course starts; that each facility has a clear indication of the learning objectives; and that a person is identified in each facility to mentor the learners. The learner's role at the hospital or clinic is to observe and evaluate the level of care provided, so that he or she has a better understanding of the role of each organization in the continuum of care and can facilitate referral of PLHA to other health providers.

Liaison with other training providers

Written arrangements need to be made with other organizations that will contribute to the training course. These could include organizations providing training in TB control, child care services, sexually transmitted infection (STI) or HIV/AIDS training.

It is essential that the organizers of the home-based care programme have a clear idea of the role and responsibilities of the caregiver so that the training programme is specifically aimed at equipping them for that role. The following is a list of the types of jobs that the caregiver can do as part of a care programme that has been planned by, or in consultation with, a doctor or registered nurse and carried out under their supervision. The list can be modified to suit the needs of the particular home-care programme.

- Promote and maintain the health of the PLHA and family.
- Provide basic information and education to PLHA, families, and the community.
- Assist the PLHA and family to identify their needs and to formulate a plan of action to address these needs.
- Promote good communication with PLHA and families.
- Use basic listening skills to provide support for the PLHA and family.
- Assist in drawing up a simple care plan to guide those who are caring for a person at home.
- Provide basic home nursing in order to alleviate pain and suffering.
- Refer the PLHA for help and advice if problems are encountered.
- Care for a dying PLHA.
- Assist and support the bereaved, including children.

The caregiver's role is limited, and he or she must liaise with qualified nursing personnel and work under their supervision and direction.

The curriculum model

Figure 3.1 shows the involvement and collaboration between the health systems, CCGs, community, PLHA, and families.

Design of a training curriculum

The course needs to provide training in the wide range of knowledge and skills that caregivers will need in order to provide a high standard of holistic care and support. Inadequate training will result in poor care. The course needs to combine theory and practice and to make provision for formative evaluation, reflective learning, and self-evaluation. The curriculum also needs to take into account the needs and resources of the home-care programme for which it is equipping caregivers.

The curriculum outlined below was developed to cater for the many different areas of home-based care. It has been divided into twelve modules, to allow

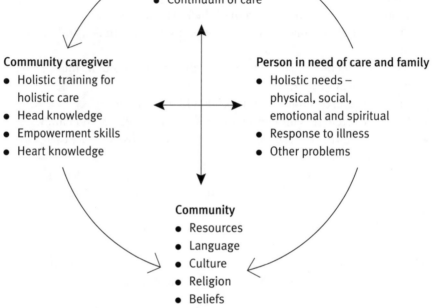

Figure 3.1 The components of a community caregiver curriculum (see Duma and Cameron 2002)

for presentation as one continuous course or for the selection of one or more modules. The learning outcomes are given here.

Module 1 - Orientation

The learner will be able to:
- demonstrate an awareness of the requirements of the course, and
- begin to develop an understanding of themselves.

The trainer will be able to:
- gain an understanding of what learners already know about HIV/AIDS or

STIs or other serious illnesses or disabilities and their attitudes to people living with the illness or disability, and
- form an idea of group dynamics and needs.

Module 2 - Community-based home caregivers

The learner will be able to:
- identify the different health care and community structures in their area
- understand their role and responsibilities in the provision of care
- explore their feelings and fears associated with their role
- record, report, and refer in an appropriate manner, and
- demonstrate an awareness of the relevant ethical/legal issues.

Module 3 - Teaching skills

The learner will be able to:
- understand their role as teachers
- use relevant teaching methods and media to teach PLHA and families, and
- identify 'teachable moments' and know how to use them.

Module 4 - Sexually transmitted infections including HIV/AIDS

The learner will be able to:
- identify the signs and symptoms of STIs
- define STIs, including HIV/AIDS
- take a history from an STI client
- explain the complications of common STIs
- explain the progression of HIV/AIDS
- discuss the causes and problems associated with STIs
- counsel STI clients on safer sexual practices, and
- explain how condoms work and demonstrate their use to a client.

Module 5 - Tuberculosis

The learner will be able to:
- identify the signs and symptoms of TB
- understand how TB is spread
- understand directly observed treatment (DOT)

- understand TB treatment, and
- understand the interaction between TB and HIV/AIDS.

Module 6 - Communication

The learner will be able to:
- understand what communication means
- identify different types of communication
- use different types of communication, and
- understand the role of communication in community entry.

Module 7 - Spiritual, religious, and cultural issues

The learner will be able to:
- describe several behaviour patterns in the community that place a person at risk of getting HIV/AIDS, STIs or TB
- discuss various barriers in the community that may prevent individuals from changing those behaviour patterns that place them at risk
- discuss the role of religion, culture, and tradition in the prevention, control, and care of HIV/AIDS, STIs or TB, and
- explain the strategies for overcoming various barriers and their implications for the prevention and control of HIV/AIDS, STIs or TB.

Module 8 - Infection control

The learner will be able to:
- define infection control
- discuss various ways infection can be spread in health care settings and communities
- describe various realistic ways and methods of preventing the spread of infections in health care settings and communities
- describe various ways of monitoring compliance and standards of practice in the prevention and control of HIV/AIDS, STIs or TB in health care/social/school settings, according to national policies
- discuss cultural practices/traditions in the community that may promote the spread of infection, and
- explain strategies that can be considered in the community for the prevention of HIV/AIDS, STIs or TB transmission.

Module 9 - Incorporating palliative care principles into basic nursing care in the home

The learner will be able to:
- identify the core elements of palliative care
- share basic knowledge of disease and disability
- discuss the importance of providing a continuum of care
- link signs and symptoms to the relevant body systems
- demonstrate efficient use of body mechanisms so as to diminish the risk of injury during the process of care
- describe appropriate interventions for common symptoms
- discuss the measures that should be taken to ensure client safety in the home
- discuss maintenance of health status for the child and adult client as well as the family
- discuss the use of 'teachable moments' in linking care to prevention
- explain when, why, and how to initiate a referral
- assess an emergency situation and provide basic life support and first aid in order to stabilize a client prior to transfer or referral
- render a wide range of basic first aid services even if the required resources have to be improvised
- maintain accurate statistics and PLHA care records
- discuss the value of evaluation and audit, and
- apply and adapt their knowledge in order to render education to the community.

Module 10 - Social support

The learner will be able to:
- define social support
- identify the beneficiaries of social support
- identify how they can benefit from social support
- identify the various needs of a PLHA and/or family
- discuss the types of social support services that can be provided
- identify the skills needed to provide social support
- identify community support and referral possibilities, and
- describe various ways of monitoring social support services.

Module 11 - Nutrition

The learner will be able to:
- identify food groups and plan suitable meals
- identify and manage problems related to nutrition
- identify dehydration and make oral rehydration solution
- teach PLHA and families how to use the available resources to grow food, and
- discuss the advantages and disadvantages of breast and bottle feeding.

Module 12 - Care of the caregiver

The learner will be able to:
- describe how they respond to their own feelings
- describe their own emotional coping mechanisms
- outline methods for measuring personal stress
- list behaviours that enhance working relationships within the team
- explain situations that may cause anxiety for health care providers in the HIV/AIDS, STIs or TB care setting, and
- describe ways of coping with situations that cause stress and anxiety for health care providers in the HIV/AIDS, STIs or TB health care setting.

Practical procedures

The following is a list of the practical procedures that the learner is expected to cover:
- washing hands
- wound dressing
- lifting
- getting PLHA out of bed
- range of motion exercises
- bathing a PLHA in bed
- shaving a male PLHA
- feeding a PLHA
- mouth care
- measuring intake/output
- breathing exercises
- helping a PLHA who is having oxygen therapy
- helping a PLHA who is coughing

- helping a PLHA who is vomiting
- collecting sputum
- taking temperature, pulse, and respiration
- demonstrating the use of male and female condoms
- putting a PLHA in the recovery position
- putting on and taking off gloves
- bed making
- positioning
- using a wheelchair
- pressure care
- washing hair in bed
- hand and foot care
- giving a bedpan
- catheter care
- testing urine
- giving medicines
- helping a PLHA who is choking
- disposing of sputum
- tepid sponging, and
- stopping bleeding.

Each learner needs to be given a booklet listing all the practical procedures in which he or she is expected to demonstrate competence. It should also have a space for learners to list visits to hospitals, clinics, or other organizations. In keeping with the principles of adult education, it is the learner's responsibility to ensure that each practical procedure is assessed and signed by a supervisor, as proof that the learner has demonstrated competence in that procedure during the training course.

Length of the course

Table 3.1 gives an indication of the time needed for each module. The time will depend on the prior knowledge of learners, the needs of the care programme for which the learners are being trained, and the size of the group (more time needs to be allocated to the evaluation of practical work for a larger group).

Table 3.1 Schedule for training

Module	Number of days required
1 Orientation	1 day
2 Community-based home caregivers	4 days, including time for community mapping
3 Teaching skills	2 days
4 Sexually transmitted infections, including HIV/AIDS	If possible, a trainer from the provincial STI or HIV/AIDS programme could be involved in this part of the course. A suggested time would be at least 3 days
5 Tuberculosis	If possible, a trainer from the provincial TB programme could be involved in this part of the course A DOTS supporter course would normally take 5 days
6 Communication	2 days Where possible, provision also needs to be made for a 5-10 day counselling course that would include pre- and post-test counselling
7 Spiritual, cultural, and religious issues	3 days
8 Infection control	2 days
9 Incorporating palliative care principles into basic nursing care in the home	This will depend on the competencies of the learners. A suggested time would be 10-15 days
10 Social support	1 day
11 Nutrition	3 days Provision also needs to be made for a visit to a food garden
12 Care of the caregiver	2 days

Table 3.1 *continued*

Practical work	This needs to be integrated with module 9
Time spent in hospital	Learners should spend an initial 1 day at each,
and clinic	followed by 5 days at the hospital later in the
	course and on-going clinic visits
Time spent at other	This will depend on the visits that can be organized.
organizations e.g.	A possible suggestion would be 3 days
old-age home,	
child centre	

Teaching methods

These should be as varied as possible and should be designed to cater for adult learners. They could include:

- lectures/discussions
- group work
- role plays
- case studies
- micro-lectures
- questionnaires, and
- stories or songs.

Assessment

In the past, on completion of training courses, many learners were given certificates of attendance. These certificates were of no real value as they gave no indication of the learner's competence in either theoretical or practical work. During any training course, provision needs to be made for on-going formative assessment of theory and practice. This is seen as an opportunity for positive feedback and as a chance to discuss and rectify problems. Time should be allocated for guidance, support, and evaluation of each learner individually. Where possible, summative evaluation at the end of the course could take the form of a two-hour written examination but, for learners who have a lower level of literacy, oral examinations should be offered. It is recommended that the pass mark for the written or oral examination be 50 per cent, and that if a learner achieves between 40 and 49 per cent, a supplementary oral examination can be given. If a learner achieves less than 40 per cent, extra guidance and support should be given before re-admission to the course is considered.

Assessment of practical work is done on an ongoing basis throughout the course as the various procedures are covered. Each learner must be able to demonstrate competence in the practical procedures and must ensure that the supervisor signs to indicate that the learner has been assessed and found to be competent.

Learner selection and interaction

Selection criteria for caregivers

The success of a home-care programme depends largely on those who are providing the day-to-day care and support, and so it is essential to have selection criteria that will guide those who are responsible for selecting learners for caregiver training. Some selection criteria could be site-specific but, as a basic guideline, caregivers should:

- have the ability to read, write, and do simple calculations (level of formal education will depend upon the area and the requirements of the programme)
- be fluent in the language of PLHA and families in the area
- show evidence of prior involvement with care programmes in the community or have a recommendation from community leaders
- be enthusiastic about working with people in need
- respect others and be committed to maintaining confidentiality
- show an interest in basic nursing care
- have good interpersonal and communication skills, and
- be committed to taking responsibility for their own learning.

Course agreement

It is strongly recommended that learners who are selected to do the training course sign an agreement with the training provider or organizers of the home-based care programme.

This needs to cover the following issues:

- the nature of the training course (it does not provide nursing training or guarantee entry into any nursing training course)
- whether or not the learners will be expected to pay course fees

- who will be responsible for transport costs, including transport to hospitals, clinics, and other organizations in the community
- the refreshments that will be provided
- dress code expected
- course attendance requirements
- assessment criteria, and
- whether or not employment will be offered to learners on successful completion of the training course.

Pre-course questionnaire and interview

It is useful to ask each applicant to complete a questionnaire that will give the selectors an idea of previous training and the reasons why the applicant is keen to do the course.

In South Africa, the National Skills Development Strategy acknowledges that prior learning needs to be recognized and taken into consideration. Figure 3.2 is an example of the type of questionnaire that could be used. Each applicant should also be given a personal interview so that verbal communication, attitude, etc. can be assessed, and so that the applicant also has the chance to ask questions about the training programme or the home-based care programme.

Conclusion

The notion of life-long learning is one of the key principles of SAQA. For many learners, caregiver training provides an opportunity for self improvement and the chance to acquire knowledge and skills that benefit others. For some, it will be the first step on a career pathway in health care, and the chance of formal employment.

Perhaps the words of two former learners convey it best:

'Thank you to train me as a home carer. I enjoy the work and I think this has now opened the door of my success.' (This young woman has gone on to complete her training as an auxiliary nurse, with distinctions in all her subjects, and is about to start her training as an enrolled nurse.)

'You make my life better. I am proud of what you taught me. We are now living the same as the others.' (This young woman is employed for the first time. She is the only breadwinner in her family and their standard of living has greatly improved.)

Community caregiver candidate questionnaire

Name:... Male/Female: ....

ID Number:.. Age (in years): ....

Address:..

.... Tel No:.....................................

....

What is the highest school standard you have passed? ....

What is your home language?...

What is the language spoken in your community? ....

Have you done any training courses in patient care? ....

If you answered Yes –

      Where did you do the course?...

      How long was the course?...

      When did you do the course?..

Have you ever taken care of a person who was very ill? ....

If you answered Yes –

      What was your relationship to the person (e.g. mother, friend)?...............

      What did you do for the person? ....

      ....

      How long did you care for him/her? ....

What would you like to learn from this course?..

....

....

Figure 3.2 Pre-course questionnaire

References

Duma, S. and S.P. Cameron. 2002. 'Home-based care training programmes for community health workers: evaluation report'. *Africa Journal of Nursing and Midwifery* 4 (1): 46–51.

Recommended reading

Ehlers, V. (ed.). 1998. *Teaching Aspects of Health Care.* Cape Town: Juta.
Evian, C. 2000. *Primary AIDS Care.* Johannesburg: Jacana Press.
Van Dyk, A. 1999. *AIDS Care and Counselling.* Cape Town: Maskew Miller Longman.

Counselling in the context of HIV/AIDS

4

Counselling in the context of HIV/AIDS

Jill Knott

Introduction

What is counselling in the setting of care for people with HIV/AIDS? HIV/AIDS has forced us all to accept a paradigm shift. This shift is from curing to caring. There is no cure for HIV/AIDS so we have no alternative but to focus our caring on the physical as well as the psychological welfare of the HIV-infected individual and his or her significant others. From the moment that an individual imagines that they might have contracted the virus, until the time of death, there is a need for psycho-social support for that person, while for that person's loved ones, support is necessary even after the death of the patient.

Counselling is a *structured* conversation, which means it is not a social conversation. *Conversation* implies a dialogue and interaction between two people; *conversation* does not imply a monologue (the kind of situation where the counsellor tells the client what to do). Counselling is also *facilitative* rather than *prescriptive*. This means that the intention of counselling is not to 'solve' everything by 'prescribing' treatment but to help or assist clients to review their problems and the options or choices they have for dealing with these problems (Egan 1990). 'Counselling should be available at all stages of the illness, from pre-test counselling to bereavement support' (van Dyk 2001, 200–1).

Phases of the counselling process

The counselling process occurs in four phases, namely:
- defining the relationship
- gathering information
- describing the problem, and
- making interventions.

These phases are generic to most therapeutic models. This division is, however, arbitrary. In practice, the phases will often overlap and interact with one another. This differentiation into phases is to provide the counsellor with a framework that might help him or her keep track of the counselling process.

Phase 1: Defining the relationship

The counsellor must clarify the counselling relationship in terms of its objectives, process, and parameters. How counsellors define themselves and the counselling context is critically important for effective and ethical counselling. Defining the relationship usually occurs in the first few moments of counselling.

Counsellors should keep the following points in mind:
- Provide a context that is unambiguously therapeutic. Establish a safe, confidential setting that clearly distinguishes the counselling relationship from social conversation.
- Provide a physical setting that is conducive to enhancing the therapeutic relationship.
- Introduce yourself and the context. Do not assume that your client knows what counselling entails. Brief the client as to the objectives and procedures of counselling and provide some idea of what is expected of the client, and what he or she may anticipate in return.
- Allow the client to negotiate the definition of the relationship by listening, observing, and confirming.
- Be sensitive to how and what you communicate. Convey the critical message of trust (i.e. that you are trustworthy), acceptance (by being non-judgemental), and structure (that you are skilled).
- Assure the client that you will maintain absolute confidentiality.
- Use the words 'HIV-positive status', conveying the words as neutrally as possible.
- Be non-judgemental.

Counselling skills that are central to this phase of counselling are:
- *Observation skills:* Distinguish between observation (what you observe) and inference (the sense you make of your observations). Inference is inevitably the cause of labelling and blaming.
- *Sensitivity to non-verbal behaviour:* (posture, direction, initiative, eye contact) – which is achieved through practising the communication skill of attentiveness.

- *Tracking skills:* Observe the client's initiatives, and connect with the client at that level. Do not follow your own agenda.
- *Responsiveness:* Be responsive to the emotional tone of the client's story. Show clients that you have understood them by reflecting their emotions in your responses.

Summary: The aim of the first phase of counselling (defining the relationship) is to establish an open relationship in which the client will feel safe enough to address personal issues and to disclose information to the counsellor.

Phase 2: Gathering information

Every conversation with a client involves some form of enquiry. During the initial interview, the counsellor spends a considerable amount of time obtaining information about the client's present circumstances so that both the client and the counsellor can understand the problem(s) and begin to think about planning possible intervention strategies. During follow-up interviews, counsellors routinely request information about attempted interventions and the events that have taken place since the previous counselling session. This phase is very important because it represents the means by which the counsellor constructs his or her understanding of the client's world. How the counsellor goes about gathering information determines what and how much she or he understands of the presenting problem. The counsellor should resist any attempt to give advice or offer quick solutions.

The gathering of information is facilitated by:

- a supportive, client-centred approach, and
- an active, benevolent curiosity or interest in the person.

Supportive, client-centred helping means that the needs of the client are central and that the ultimate purpose of the process is to identify and implement actions that will improve the client's situation (Egan 1990). It is, therefore, important to allow clients to tell their stories in their own way. Client-centred helping is most clearly evident in counselling techniques such as basic empathy, advanced empathy, self-disclosure, and immediacy.

Active benevolent curiosity relies on the counsellor's observation and questioning. By using active listening techniques and communication skills, the counsellor tries to gain an accurate understanding of the client's problems, the way in which he or she is experiencing these problems, and what the client needs for a better future. The counsellor should keep the following points in mind when he or she interviews clients:

- Learn and adopt the client's language.
- Use open, not closed questions.
- Be sensitive to feedback about specific content.
- Be respectful.
- Be patient and revisit topics if it is necessary to do so.
- Avoid suggesting solutions and prescriptions.
- Deal with multiple levels of understanding (content, emotions, behaviour, and cognition).
- Involve context in your enquiry.
- Focus on process over time. Understand and recognize patterns and trends.

Summary: The primary purpose of the information-gathering phase is to make the counsellor an 'expert' on the client's context and his or her response to HIV/AIDS, by learning from the client about his or her situation.

Phase 3: Describing the problem dynamic

Once the counsellor has dealt with the information-gathering phase, he or she needs to articulate his or her understanding of the problem dynamic on the basis of that information.

The first formal intervention the counsellor should make is to describe his or her understanding of the problem. All clients, but especially HIV-infected clients, are entitled to know what the counsellor thinks. By sharing their knowledge, counsellors allow their clients to resolve personal issues autonomously. By not describing this understanding, the counsellor introduces a power-political dimension. This power-political dimension means the counsellor uses his or her expertise, experience, and (secret) superior knowledge to control and manipulate the client. Such an approach obviously constitutes an implicit but serious breach of ethics.

The following guidelines will help the counsellor to describe the problem dynamics:

- Introduce the phase and focus attention on what you are about to say.
- Be concise but comprehensive in your descriptions.
- Use culturally and developmentally appropriate language (the client must be able to understand you).

- Never blame or judge.
- Include significant others in your descriptions.
- Focus on relationships rather than individual attributes.

With experience, the counsellor will find that clients often blame themselves for the way they feel or even for their illness. They might also feel sad or even angry. Just hearing from the counsellor that these feelings are understandable, may lessen the feeling of isolation in the person.

Summary: Describing the problem dynamic is an attempt to articulate aspects of the client's experience in such a way that they are recognizable and confirming, but in a sense that is novel to the client. This phase focuses on facilitating self-exploration, clarifying feelings, and describing the problem in such a way that interventions can be planned.

Phase 4: Intervention or action

Intervention is not a solution. It is a process in which the client becomes involved in order to improve the quality of his or her life. In addition to providing supportive client-centred counselling, the counsellor also acts as an active agent of change. The aim is to give the client the opportunity to resolve personal issues about his or her HIV-positive status in a safe environment. In this process, the counsellor will use a number of non-directive counselling techniques such as basic empathy, advanced empathy, self-disclosure, immediacy, reflection, and interpretation. Showing that you understand feelings and reactions, and that you respect the person without judgement, is already 'doing something'.

Directive counselling is often helpful in those cases where the focus should be on practical, accessible aspects of the client's response to HIV/AIDS (e.g. safer sex practices).

In order to be directive in HIV/AIDS counselling, the counsellor needs to have the following skills:

- a good working knowledge of HIV infection and AIDS and the ability and interest to keep abreast of developments in this rapidly changing field
- the ability to communicate information in an accurate, consistent, and objective manner, and
- the ability to feel comfortable when speaking to people about sexuality and sex (if the counsellor feels embarrassed to talk about sex, the client will not feel free to discuss sex).

Summary: The focus in the intervention or action phase moves from the identification and description of problems to setting goals that are aimed at resolving the problem, deciding on methods of achieving them, and monitoring and evaluating the results.

Values underlying the counselling process

The counsellor's values and attitudes play a critical role in the helping process. The way counsellors see themselves and their clients, the helping process, and the world around them, will affect the way in which they counsel.

Counsellors should enter the helping process with sincere respect for their clients, an open and genuine attitude, and the intention of helping their clients to empower themselves and take responsibility for their own lives.

Important values are:

- respect
- genuineness or congruence
- empowerment and self-responsibility, and
- confidentiality.

Respect

Respect is an attitude that portrays the belief that every person is a worthy being who is competent to decide what he or she really wants from life. A counsellor can show respect for the client in the following ways:

- Accept the client by showing unconditional positive regard, i.e. you accept the person irrespective of their values or behaviour.
- Respect the client's rights, i.e. their right to their own feelings, beliefs, opinions, and choices.
- Respect the uniqueness of each client.
- Refrain from judgement.
- Remain serene and imperturbable.
- Show respect that is both considerate and tough-minded.
- Acknowledge the person's diversity, their culture, ethnicity, spirituality, sexual orientation, family, educational, and socio-economic status. Avoid stereotyping, and respect people's traditions and customs.

Genuineness or congruence

A congruent person is honest and transparent in the counselling relationship because he or she surrenders all roles and facades. A genuine, congruent counsellor demonstrates the following values and behaviours:

- Be yourself: sincere, honest, and clear.
- Be honest with yourself and your clients.
- Do not over-emphasize the helping role.
- Do not patronize or condescend.
- Keep the client's agenda in focus.
- Do not be defensive.

Empowerment and self-responsibility

The empowerment of clients should be based on the following values (Egan 1990, 52–3):

- Believe in your client's pursuit of growth, self-actualization, and self-determination. See this from the client's frame of reference and accept that you, as a counsellor, cannot decide what a client's goals would be or what would be best for him or her. Accept the principle that the client knows himself or herself better than anyone else and that he or she is in the best position to explore, expose, and understand the self.
- Believe in the clients' ability to change if they choose to do so. The counsellor's basic attitude should be that the clients have the resources both to participate in the counselling process and to manage their lives more effectively. Since these resources may be blocked or disabled in a variety of ways, it is the task of the counsellor to help clients identify, free, and utilize these resources.
- Refrain from rescuing the client. Rescuing reflects the rescuer's needs. It is typically motivated by needs such as a lack of confidence in the capability of the person being rescued, a need to feel important, or a need to be needed.
- Share the helping process with clients.
- Help clients to see that the counselling sessions are work sessions.
- Help clients become better problem-solvers.

Confidentiality

Confidentiality in a counselling context is non-negotiable. A counsellor may under no circumstances disclose HIV status or any information to anybody without the express permission of the client.

Confidentiality in the HIV/AIDS field is difficult and complex. Is one's responsibility to the client, their partner, or the community at large? And how does one come to terms with some of the moral issues that the virus and its spread evoke?

Basic communication skills for counselling

As a counsellor, one needs basic communication skills to be able to facilitate change. These skills include attending, listening, basic empathy, probing, and summarizing, and are all essential tools for both relationship building and constructive change (Egan 1990).

Attending

Attending refers to the ways in which counsellors can be with their clients both physically and psychologically (Egan 1990). Effective attending tells clients that you are with them and they can share their world with you.

There are certain micro-skills that counsellors can use when attending to their clients, and Egan (1990, 63–4) summarizes these skills under the acronym 'SOLER':

S Face the client *squarely*. Adopt a posture that indicates involvement.

O Adopt an *open posture*. Crossed arms and legs may show diminished involvement.

L *Lean* towards the client (when appropriate). Read the client's body language.

E Maintain good *eye contact* but do not stare. Be aware that direct eye contact is not acceptable in all cultures.

R Try to be *relaxed* and natural.

Effective attending puts counsellors in a position to listen carefully.

Listening

Listening refers to the ability of counsellors to capture and understand the messages clients communicate as they tell their stories.

According to Egan (1990), active listening involves four skills:

- *Listening to understand the client's verbal messages.* The counsellor needs to listen to the mix of experiences, behaviour, and feelings that the client uses to describe his or her situation.

- *Listening to and interpreting the client's non-verbal messages.* Non-verbal messages include bodily behaviour (posture, body movement, and gestures), facial expressions (smiles, frowns, raised eyebrows, twisted lips, grimaces), voice-related behaviour (tone, pitch, voice-level, intensity), observable physiological responses (quickened breathing, blushing, paleness, pupil dilation), and general appearance (grooming and dress).
- *Listen to and understand in context.* People are more than the sum of their verbal messages. The person needs to be seen as a whole in their social context.
- *Listen with empathy.* Empathetic counselling requires helpers to put their own concerns aside and be fully 'with' the client.

Listening is not an easy skill to acquire. Counsellors should be aware of the following hindrances to effective listening (Egan 1990):
- inadequate listening (it is easy to be distracted and lose track of what is being said)
- evaluative listening (the counsellor judges and labels the client as he or she speaks)
- filtered listening (we tend to listen to ourselves, other people, and the world around us through biase [often prejudiced] filters; Filtered listening distorts our understanding of our clients)
- labels as filters, i.e. 'that woman with AIDS'
- fact-centred rather than person-centred listening, i.e. asking only factual questions
- rehearsing, i.e. thinking of what you will say next, and
- sympathetic listening (to sympathize with someone is to become that person's 'accomplice'; sympathy conveys pity).

Basic empathy

Empathy is the ability to recognize and acknowledge the feelings of another person without experiencing those same emotions – it is an attempt to understand the world of the client by temporarily 'stepping into his or her shoes'. This understanding of the client's world must then be shared with the client in a verbal or non-verbal way.

The key elements of basic empathy are as follows:
- *Formula for basic empathy:* Basic empathy can be expressed in the following formula: You feel … (name the relevant emotion expressed by the client) …

because … (or when) … (indicates the relevant experiences and behaviours that gave rise to the feelings).

- *Experiences, behaviours, and feelings as elements of empathy:* An empathetic response has the same key elements as the client's story, namely experiences, behaviour, and feelings. The counsellor should respond to the client's feelings by referring to the correct family of emotions and by referring to the correct intensity of emotions. Egan named four main families of emotions, namely sad, mad, bad, and glad. Fear can also be included. Nonverbals are also important ways of conveying emotions.

Note the following hints for communicating empathy:
- Give yourself time to think.
- Use short responses.
- Gear your response to the client, but remain yourself.

Probing or questioning

Probing involves statements and questions from the counsellor that enable clients to explore more fully any relevant issues in their lives (Egan 1990). Probes can take the form of statements, questions, requests, single words or phrases, and non-verbal prompts. Egan (1990) gives the following advice about probes. Probes serve the following purposes:
- to encourage non-assertive or reluctant clients to tell their stories
- to help clients to remain focused on relevant and important issues
- to help clients to identify experiences, behaviours, and feelings that give a fuller picture to their story; in other words, to fill in the missing pieces of the picture
- to help clients to move forward in the helping process, and
- to help clients understand themselves and their problem situations more fully.

Summarizing

Summarizing serves the purpose of focusing on what has happened in a session and sometimes is a challenge to the client and assists with moving forward.

Summarizing is appropriate:
- when you are beginning a new session, since summary at this point can give

direction to clients who do not know where to start and can also prevent clients from repeating what they have already said

- when a session seems to be going nowhere, and
- when a client gets stuck.

Counselling in a multi-cultural society

For a century or more, indigenous or traditional African healing and modern Western forms of counselling and psychotherapy operated side by side – in almost mutual isolation.

Although traditional healing and Western counselling are based on different philosophical assumptions, there are certain similarities that are universal to counselling. There are also many differences that need to be taken into account.

Differences between traditional African and Western beliefs and assumptions

Traditional African thought is characterized by a holistic outlook. The traditional African approach integrates the biological, psycho-social, and trans-personal aspects of illness. African people do not necessarily distinguish between physical and mental illness. They see illness as affecting the whole human being – including a person's relationship with his or her ancestors and the community. They believe that physical, mental, and social systems are interconnected and that changes in one system inevitably affect changes in the other.

Another important difference is the value placed on the group rather than on the individual, in African culture. In the African tradition, people do not generate knowledge by introspectively examining their own feelings, their own thinking, or their own intelligence (the ancient Western tradition of self-analysis). Africans acquire knowledge from their relationships with the sky, the land, their families, their communities, and their ancestors (Beuster 1997; Buhrman 1986; Hammond-Tooke 1989; Mbiti 1969).

Western societies, however, believe in individualism and the rights of the individual. This emphasizes personal autonomy and individual initiative. There is also a tendency for Western counsellors to over-emphasize the rational, logical, and intellectual, while neglecting the unconscious, intuitive, and trans-personal sides of the psyche (Beuster 1997; Bodibe and Sodi 1997).

Similarities and differences between traditional African healing and Western counselling

There are the following similarities and differences between traditional healing and Western psychotherapy or counselling.

Similarities

Both traditional healing and Western psychotherapy or counselling:
- emphasize the importance of building a relationship that is based on trust
- aim at personality integration and positive growth
- emphasize the expression of feelings (although ways of expressing feelings differ), and
- rely on communication skills.

Differences

Traditional healing and Western psychotherapy or counselling differ in that:
- an African approach is symbolic, intuitive, and integrally part of traditional African beliefs and cosmology, while Western counselling is based largely on scientific, logical principles, which have no direct link to symbolism
- the traditional healer explores the client's relationships with his or her ancestors and neighbours, because conspiracies with witches and sorcerers can cause problems, and
- traditionally, it is important to sort out things between the client and the ancestors, while Western counsellors concentrate on the exploration of feelings and the promotion of insight and problem solutions.

General cultural considerations

Counsellors should bear the following general cultural considerations in mind:
- When counselling cross-culturally, be very careful to avoid being seen as condescending or patronizing.
- Explore and acknowledge your own prejudices, stereotyping, and cultural assumptions.
- Recognize the limitations that cross-cultural counselling imposes.

Language barriers

The use of an interpreter can cause problems. Translators often translate according to their own personal frame of reference. Keep the following precautions in mind when using an interpreter (Whaley and Wong 1999):

- Using a child as a translator is considered an insult to adults.
- If the client and interpreter are of different cultures, this could create difficulties.
- Confidentiality is a problem.
- Ensure that the client fully understands what is being said.
- Ask one question at a time.

Different HIV counselling programmes and services

HIV counselling can be long term or short term and has two general aims, namely:

- the prevention of HIV transmission, and
- the support of those affected directly and indirectly by HIV.

It is important that counselling should have the dual aims of prevention and support, because the spread of HIV can be prevented by changes in behaviour. Behavioural change can be assisted by one-to-one prevention counselling, particularly where the possibility for discussion elsewhere may be undermined by the force of social stigma. When patients know that they have HIV infection or disease, they can suffer great psycho-social and psychological stresses through a fear of social stigma and rejection, a fear of disease progression, and the uncertainties connected with future management of HIV.

The HIV pandemic, more than any other, has brought with it the need for health care workers to have counselling skills. The life-changing nature of an HIV diagnosis requires that all persons be fully informed of the consequences of a positive result before they are tested (pre-test counselling), and thereafter that they be told the result and given support if it is positive (post-test counselling). There are a number of other situations in the context of HIV where counselling is required, for example bereavement counselling for individual family members and also for children infected with and affected by HIV/AIDS. It is, therefore, important for health care professionals to develop some personal basic counselling skills.

Aims of HIV counselling

HIV counselling aims to:
- provide a supportive environment
- help clients manage problems and issues
- explore coping skills they have used before and develop new ones
- empower clients to become self-sufficient in dealing with emerging issues and problems
- counsel HIV-negative clients so that they know how to remain negative
- counsel HIV-positive clients on how to avoid cross-infection and how to prevent infecting others, and
- explore options with the client that will help her or him to bring about necessary changes in behaviour. These options should include abstinence, monogamy (mutual faithfulness), and the correct use of condoms.

The Health Professions Council of South Africa and the South African Medical Association recommend that since an HIV test interferes with a person's right to freedom and security of person and privacy, a person may only be tested:
- at his or her own request
- after he or she has given informed consent, preferably written, or
- when otherwise authorized by legislation or a court order.

The issue of informed consent is a very important one. Informed consent is based on the assessment of two conditions. These are an assessment of the patient's competence to decide, and his or her voluntariness or degree of separation from other coercive influences that will compromise the voluntary character of consent. Informal consent can be seen as a very active part of the doctor-patient relationship. Far from being a mere legal notion, static or situational, it carries great moral significance, and impacts greatly upon the day-to-day management of the disease.

Before testing, the health professional should:
- check for legislative processes that may regulate HIV testing for insurance policies, for instance, and in places like prisons, schools, the workplace, etc.
- confirm there is a clinical indication
- ensure that pre-test counselling has been done adequately or do so personally
- ensure that the client has been fully informed and therefore consented, and
- be in a position to ensure confidentiality.

Pre-test counselling – important checklist

The counsellor should note the following:

- Assure the client that both counselling and testing are confidential procedures.
- Be sure that if more than one session is required, it can be offered.
- Provide information about HIV infection and transmission and its links to AIDS, sexually transmitted infections, and TB.
- Provide information on the technical aspects of testing and its implications and the meaning of the terms 'positive' and 'negative', and the window period.
- Discuss the implications of a positive or negative diagnosis.
- Provide information about the client's legal rights in terms of who to tell (sexual partner/s) or not to tell (for example, the employer, third parties, etc.). Clients are not obliged to tell anyone apart from their sexual partners. (*The Promotion of Access to Information Act* of 2000 came into operation in March 2002, and details procedures that give effect to the human right to information. This could affect a person's ability to get information about an individual's physical condition and could perhaps enable a person to get information about someone's HIV status.)
- Evaluate risk behaviour. Find out why the individual wants to be tested and the nature and extent of previous and present high-risk behaviour. Discuss the steps they should take to prevent future infection or transmission.
- Determine the client's coping resources and support systems in the event of a positive result.
- Contain the client's emotions as they deal with issues about relationships.
- Determine whether the client wishes to be tested immediately.
- Assure the client that you will respect their decision.
- Provide a sense of support for the client.

Post-test counselling

Post-test counselling helps the client to work through the crisis and other issues that might arise as a result of being told their HIV status.

Counselling skills needed during the post-test counselling session are:

- empathy
- non-judgemental approach
- active listening
- clear discussion and information giving

- appropriate use of health education material
- ability to develop an appropriate rapport
- facilitating appropriate planning by enabling client decision making, and
- motivating appropriate self-care and reflection.

Giving the results

The following are important points to bear in mind when giving the results:

- Give the results as soon as they are received. Give the results simply and in person. The results should never be given over the telephone.
- The same person who did the pre-test counselling should, if possible, give the results and do post-test counselling. The continuity is important.
- If possible, make sure the client will be supported once they leave your office.

If the HIV result is negative:

- Discuss the window period.
- Reinforce the message of prevention and safer sexual practices.
- Pick up on issues raised in the pre-test counselling session.
- Discuss referral for ongoing counselling, especially if there are ongoing risk factors.

HIV-positive result

A person who has tested HIV-positive may never have the same quality of life again. They will need to reassess their lives and how they will live their lives. At the initial interview, when the client is given the news of her or his positive HIV status, they may be too shocked to absorb much of what they are told. Therefore, it is initially important to:

- concentrate on managing the resultant crisis and address the client's immediate concerns, and
- be careful of information overload in the first session.

Later (often during a second counselling session):

- continue to contain emotions
- answer any questions
- remind the client that a partner needs to know her or his partner's HIV status

- discuss who they will tell
- discuss medical assistance and where to get it
- discuss safer sex
- discuss the cost and availability of antiretroviral therapies (ART) and drug trials
- discuss the importance of a healthy lifestyle (food, rest, and exercise), and
- explore the need to eliminate alcohol, smoking, or drugs.

Ongoing counselling helps the client to deal with issues such as partner notification, relationship difficulties, queries about health and treatment, as well as disclosure to others. Counselling support should be available to the client in the weeks and months following the positive test result. Being identified HIV-positive may require constructive planning for the future, such as deciding on the future welfare and care of children.

Ongoing counselling involves understanding a person in their social and familial contexts and many patients derive crucial support from parents and friends.

Good, early intervention can help the individual to cope well in the months and years to come. It will encourage wider medical care and intervention, and will provide psycho-social support when necessary.

Symptomatic HIV infection/diagnosis of AIDS

Most patients will remain well and asymptomatic for years after their initial infection with HIV. However, the onset of HIV-related symptoms, some of which may be classified as an AIDS diagnosis, can precipitate a psychological crisis. Many patients who have remained well, believe the illness is not going to happen to them and the resulting shock can bring back many of the issues raised at the HIV diagnosis. In this instance, the aim of counselling is to assist the patient in adjustment and to be alert to the need for redefining support, particularly in relation to community-based services such as home-care teams.

Crisis intervention

Crisis intervention is a form of emotional 'first aid' or a short-term helping process designed to provide immediate relief in an emergency situation. Crisis intervention is active, direct, and brief and occurs shortly after a crisis has occurred. Gilliland and James (2001) propose a six-step model of crisis intervention.

This is an action-oriented, situationally-based method of crisis intervention. Because of the nature of the HIV/AIDS illness, there are often crises that arise in the life of the person living with the virus. These could include the initial HIV diagnosis and would also occur at the time of an AIDS diagnosis. As the various opportunistic illnesses affect the person, each one could constitute a crisis situation.

The entire six-step process is carried out under an umbrella of assessment by the counsellor. The first three steps of (1) defining the problem, (2) ensuring client safety, and (3) providing support, are more listening activities than they are actions. The final three steps of (4) examining alternatives, (5) making plans, and (6) obtaining commitment to positive action, are largely action behaviours on the part of the counsellor, even though listening is always present along with assessment.

Step 1: Defining the problem

The first step in crisis intervention is to define and understand the problem from the client's point of view. To do this, the counsellor needs to use the skills of empathy, genuineness, acceptance, and positive regard.

Step 2: Ensuring client safety

Client safety can be defined as minimizing the physical and psychological danger to self and others.

Step 3: Providing support

The counsellor needs to show the client that he or she is valued and important, and to do this the counsellor needs to show total acceptance and unconditional positive regard for the individual, regardless of the circumstances of the crisis.

Step 4: Examining alternatives

Step 4 in crisis intervention addresses an area that both clients and counsellors often neglect – exploring a wide array of appropriate choices available to the client. Some clients in crisis believe there are no options. Clients can be made aware that there are alternatives. These alternatives can be divided into the following:

- *situational supports,* i.e. people who know the client and care about his or her welfare
- *coping mechanisms* are those actions, behaviours, or environmental resources that the client might use to help get through the present crisis, and
- *positive and constructive thinking patterns* on the part of the client are ways of thinking that might substantially alter the client's view of the problem and lessen the client's level of stress and anxiety.

Clients experiencing crisis do not need a lot of choices, they need appropriate choices that are realistic for their situation.

Step 5: Making plans

Step 5 flows logically from Step 4 – a plan should include the following:
- Identify additional persons, groups, and other referral sources that can be contacted for immediate support.
- Provide coping mechanisms – something concrete and positive for the client to do now; definite action steps that the client can own and comprehend.
- Focus on systematic problem solving for the client. The critical element in developing a plan is that clients do not feel robbed of their power, independence, and self-respect. The central issues in planning are the client's control and autonomy.

Step 6: Obtaining commitment

Often the commitment step simply involves asking the client to verbally summarize the plan. During this step, do not forget all the other helping steps and skills such as assessing, ensuring safety, and providing support. The core listening skills are as important to the commitment step as they are to the problem definition or any other step.

Assessing is an integral part of each of the six steps and enables the counsellor to:
- determine the severity of the crisis
- determine the client's current emotional status – the client's level of emotional mobility or immobility

- determine the alternatives, coping mechanisms, support systems, or other resources available to the client, and
- determine the client's attitude towards suicide.

Summary

The six steps in crisis intervention serve to organize and simplify the work of the crisis counsellor. Step 1 explores and defines the problem from the client's point of view. Step 2 ensures the client's physical and psychological safety. Step 3 provides support for the person in crisis. Step 4 examines alternatives available to the client. Step 5 assists the client in developing a plan of action. Finally, Step 6 helps the client to make a commitment to carry out a definite action plan.

Assessment of the person and the crisis situation is the keystone for initiating intervention. Assessment techniques, such as evaluating the severity of the crisis; appraising the client's thinking, feeling, emotions and behaviour patterns; assessing the seriousness and possible suicidal tendencies of the client; looking into the client's background for contributing factors; evaluating the client's resources, coping mechanisms, and support systems are presented and explored.

Listening is a fundamental imperative for all successful counselling, including crisis intervention. People need to be encouraged to take an active part in planning their own care. Such an approach includes encouraging problem-solving, participation in treatment, decision making, active distractions through recreation and socializing, and emphasizing self-worth and the potential for personal control over manageable issues in life. Finally, the value of groups in HIV psycho-social and stress management is amply demonstrated. Groups are valuable in reducing an individual's sense of isolation – of being the only one – and in providing a safe place to express feelings, to share experiences, and to learn successful coping styles from others. Groups have a very constructive social support function and may help in risk reduction by establishing and emphasizing an ethos of safer sex or safer intravenous drug use, for instance.

To date, studies have shown the value of groups in stress management with gay men, with sharing coping experiences with people with HIV, and with managing AIDS-related bereavement.

Bereavement counselling

There are two distinct types of bereavement that one deals with when discussing bereavement in terms of HIV/AIDS. The first is the anticipatory grief and loss that the person experiences when told he or she has full-blown AIDS. The second is bereavement after a death. HIV-infected people often suffer from the following psycho-social, spiritual, and socio-economic experiences and needs (van Dyk, 2001):

- *Fear:* HIV-infected individuals have many fears. They fear being stigmatized, isolated, and rejected. They fear the uncertainty of the future, i.e. will there be pain and disfigurement, who will look after them? Many HIV-infected individuals have experienced the pain and death of loved ones and friends who have already died of AIDS and they know and fear what awaits them.

- *Loss:* HIV-infected people often feel that they have lost everything that is most important to them. They experience loss of control, loss of anatomy, loss of their ambitions and their physical attractiveness, loss of sexual relationships, status and respect in the community, financial stability, and independence. They fear the loss of their ability to care for themselves and their families and they fear the loss of their jobs, their friends, and their family. They mourn the loss of life itself. HIV-infected people also feel they have lost their privacy and their control over their lives once they begin to need constant care. They lose confidence in themselves and suffer a loss of self-esteem and self-worth occasioned by the rejection of people who are important to them.

- *Grief:* People with HIV infection grieve all the above losses and also experience anticipatory grief in respect of their own death.

- *Guilt:* People infected with HIV express guilt and self-reproach for having contracted HIV and for also having possibly infected others. Feelings of guilt may be associated with being homosexual or with sexuality in general.

- *Denial:* Most HIV-positive people go through a phase of denial. Denial is an important defence mechanism and can reduce emotional stress. If denial causes destructive behaviour, such as refusing appropriate medical care or continued indulgence in unrestrained high-risk behaviour, it can be seen as being destructive.

- *Anger:* HIV-infected people are often angry at themselves and angry at the world in general. They are angry as there is no cure for AIDS and the future is so uncertain.

- *Anxiety:* The chronic uncertainty associated with the progress of HIV infection often aggravates feelings of anxiety. The risk of infecting others can change lifestyles radically.

- *Depression:* HIV-infected individuals often suffer from depression because of the multiple losses they experience in their lives. It is important to recognize the symptoms of depression and refer appropriately.

- *Suicidal thinking:* Anger directed inwards may manifest as self-blame, self-destructive behaviour, or suicidal impulses or intention. The suicide rate among HIV-infected individuals is higher than in the general population.
- *Socio-economic issues:* HIV-infected individuals face the loss of a job and income, discrimination, social stigma, relationship changes and changing requirements for sexual expression, financial problems, and inability to afford expensive drugs or lifesaving treatment.
- *AIDS dementia:* Another really important loss experienced by the AIDS patient is the onset of AIDS Dementia Complex (ADC). Family and friends may describe a sense that the patient has 'changed' in ways that are subtle, but important. They may feel that the patient is less interested in those things that used to be of great interest, they may be less talkative, less 'sharp'. The patients themselves will complain that they think more slowly and have difficulty in completing and carrying out tasks. They may report balance and coordination problems. Behavioural changes such as social withdrawal and slowness of speech and movement may also be observed.

During this stage, the individual with ADC can participate actively in treatment and management decisions and should be encouraged to do so. The intervention strategy at this stage should be to help the patient learn to adapt to changing abilities by learning to compensate for any deficiencies.

As the disease progresses and cognitive skills continue to decline, the ability to make reasonable judgements becomes increasingly impaired. Frequent periods of disorientation can occur. These patients develop severe attention-deficit disorders and are often unable to follow conversations. Once this degree of disability is reached, the individual has lost the means to learn how to adapt creatively to the disability.

Caring for the individual with AIDS who develops dementia can be an overwhelming and burdensome experience. Family members and partners face caring for someone with a terminal illness who is experiencing increasing physical debilitations, as well as deteriorating cognitive abilities, personality changes, and increasing financial responsibilities. Caregivers may feel that their need to settle unresolved issues or to complete their 'final goodbyes' is thwarted by the patient's dementia.

HIV-related cognitive impairment and ADC are frightening possibilities for those who are infected and those who care about them. Dementia causes additional problems and stresses for all involved and carers, as well as patients, need help and support. Counselling should be very supportive.

Having considered the losses, grief, and despair experienced by the patient with HIV/AIDS, one can look at the grief and bereavement experienced by the family, friends, and lovers who survive the death of a loved one from HIV/AIDS. One can start by looking at a few definitions:

- *Grief* is the emotional response to the event.
- *Mourning* is the cultural process.
- *Bereavement* is an event.

Losing a significant other to death is considered one of the most stressful events in a person's life and, even in the most uncomplicated circumstances, the psychological tasks of grief work present the survivor with multiple challenges. The loss of someone from AIDS can be especially difficult, and the subsequent bereavement process can become complicated.

Normal grief

Bereavement, or the state of grieving that accompanies a loss, is not an illness, it is a natural, healthy response. Bereavement is experienced in all cultures, observed in many species of animals, and can result in a broad range of physical and emotional symptoms. No one will necessarily experience all of them, nor must all be present for grief to be considered normal. However, understanding that many kinds of feelings are to be expected, can make the experience of grief much more manageable.

When loss occurs, usual patterns of routine behaviour are disrupted. People stop doing things they ordinarily do. Studies have shown that acute grief constitutes a definite syndrome, with both psychological and somatic symptomatology. The signs of grief may either appear immediately or be delayed; they may even appear to be absent. Symptoms may be distorted, exaggerated, or highly variable and will differ among individuals and according to different circumstances.

Grief affects a person socially, emotionally, spiritually, physically, and behaviourally and can produce both positive and negative states. The range of somatic symptoms that may occur in normal grief include tightness of throat, choking, shortness of breath, sighing, an empty feeling in the abdomen, a pain in the chest, chills, and tremors. These bodily sensations may be accompanied by intense mental distress, tension, loneliness, and anguish. The bereaved person's perception may also become disorganized to such a degree that events seem unreal.

Survivors describe periods of hallucinations or euphoria. People may have heightened perceptual and emotional sensitivity to persons and events in the immediate environment and may be preoccupied with images of the deceased. Hostility, irritability, and a feeling of general restlessness are common. Sometimes the bereaved talk incessantly about the deceased, sometimes they never talk about the person who died.

Other commonly experienced feelings indicate guilt or anger in addition to sadness, longing, loneliness, and sorrow. Grief produces feelings of anger and outrage at the injustice of the loss and frustration and a sense of impotence at the inability to control events.

Elizabeth Kubler-Ross (1989) is one of the founders in the field of writing on death and dying. According to Kubler-Ross (1989), patients go through five stages when approaching death and dying. These stages are denial, anger, bargaining, depression, and acceptance. She also feels that bereaved people go through these same stages. Kubler-Ross's stages must not be seen as a linear, step-by-step guide, but rather as the stages for different periods of time. They may replace each other, and they may even exist together.

There are many different theories around grief and bereavement, but the one I will describe here is the theory put forward by J. William Worden in his book *Grief Counselling and Grief Therapy* (1991).

Attachment theory

Before one can fully comprehend the impact of a loss and the human behaviour associated with it, one must have some understanding of the meaning of attachment.

One of the key figures and primary thinkers in this area is British psychiatrist John Bowlby. To develop his themes, Bowlby (1969, 1977) has included data from ethnology, control theory, cognitive psychology, neurophysiology, and developmental biology. Bowlby does not believe that attachment bonds between individuals develop only in order to have certain biological drives met. He believes that these attachments come from a need for security and safety and develop early in life and are usually directed toward a few specific individuals and tend to endure throughout a large part of the life cycle (Bowlby, 1969).

If the goal of attachment behaviour is to maintain an affectionate bond, situations that endanger this bond give rise to certain very specific reactions. The greater the potential for loss, the more intense these reactions can be. There is evidence that all humans grieve a loss to some degree or other. Worden (1991) believes that there are four tasks of mourning. These are as follows:

Task 1: To accept the reality of the loss. The first task of grieving is to come fully face to face with the reality that the person is dead, that the person is gone and will not return. People might deny that the death has occurred and this denial can be a protection against the pain of the loss.

Task 2: To work through the pain of grief. The various experts in grief and bereavement such as Parkes, Bowlby, Stroebe, and Silverman, all stress the importance of bereaved people working through the pain of grief. This pain can be physical, emotional, or behavioural. If it is necessary for the bereaved person to go through the pain of grief, what happens if this does not occur? John Bowlby (1977) has said that people who avoid all conscious grieving will eventually break down – usually with some form of depression. One of the aims of grief counselling is to help facilitate this difficult second task, so that they do not carry the pain with them throughout their lives.

Task 3: To adjust to the environment from which the deceased is missing. Adjusting to a new environment means different things to different people, depending on what the relationship was with the deceased and the various roles the deceased played. The survivors are not usually aware of all the roles played by the deceased until some time has elapsed after the death.

Many survivors resent having to learn new skills and to take on roles themselves that were formerly performed by their partners. Bereaved people also have to adjust to their own sense of self, i.e. 'Who am I without the person who has died?'

Bereavement can lead to depression: bereaved people see themselves as helpless, inadequate, incapable, childlike, or personally bankrupt. However, over time these negative images usually give way to more positive ones. One's sense of the world can change, as can one's fundamental life values and philosophical beliefs – beliefs that are influenced by our families, peers, education, and religion, as well as life experiences. It is not unusual for the bereaved to feel they have lost direction in life.

Task 4: To emotionally relocate the deceased and move on with life. The counsellor's task here is to help the bereaved find an appropriate place for the dead in their emotional lives – a place that will enable them to go on living effectively in the world. The fourth task is hindered by holding on to the past attachment rather than going on and forming new ones. Some people find loss so painful that they make a pact never to love again. This can be a very difficult task for people and they often feel guilty at the thought of getting on with their lives.

In Worden's (1991) view, mourning is finished when the four tasks of mourning are accomplished. It is impossible to set a definitive date for this, yet, within the bereavement literature, there are all sorts of attempts to set dates – four months, one year, two years, never. With the loss of someone really close, two years is not too long.

Useful techniques in counselling

Some useful techniques in counselling are:
- Evocative language: Using the words 'death and dying' can help people with reality issues.
- Use of symbols: Have the bereaved person bring in photographs of the deceased person.
- Writing: Write letters to the deceased to perhaps complete 'unfinished business'. Keep a diary or a journal to record thoughts, feelings, and dreams.
- Drawing: It can help people who have difficulties expressing feelings to put them down on paper.

Grieving special types of loss

Suicide

A family member who is grieving for someone who has committed suicide is not only left with a sense of loss, they are left with a legacy of shame, fear, rejection, anger, and guilt. Shame is a very specific feeling with which survivors of a suicide are left. People avoid them and they avoid people. Often other people do not discuss the death.

Guilt is another common feeling. People have a feeling that they should or could have done something to prevent the death. Guilt can sometimes manifest as blame. Some people handle their own sense of culpability by projecting their guilt onto others and blaming them for the death.

Anger is also very prevalent in the feelings experienced by the survivors of suicide.

Sudden death

There are certain special features that should be considered when working with the survivors of sudden death. Sudden deaths could perhaps evoke the following responses:

- a sense of unreality (shock is greater)
- nightmares and intrusive images
- guilt feelings
- the need to blame someone for the death
- frequent involvement of medical and legal authorities (getting on with the tasks of mourning is difficult [if not impossible] until the legal aspects of the case are resolved), and
- a sense of helplessness; the survivors feel they have lost control of their world, their world becomes unsafe; people become very agitated and feel helpless.

Crisis intervention techniques are highly effective when helping people cope with sudden death.

The final type of grief that needs to be discussed is anticipatory grief. The term 'anticipatory grief' refers to the grieving that occurs prior to the actual loss. In this type of situation, the mourning process begins early and involves the tasks of mourning already discussed.

AIDS bereavement

The bereavement process for AIDS-related deaths is complicated by a number of special issues in addition to those commonly raised by the grieving of any loss. While AIDS bereavement can, and often does, follow all the stages of normal grief, these special features make the possibility of complicated bereavement more likely, and the need for special interventions with these individuals more important.

Factors that differentiate AIDS bereavement from other kinds of grief are as follows:

Stigma: Whether one has lost a spouse, a lover, a child, a sibling, or a friend, grieving an AIDS death includes some degree of stigma. The disease draws attention to a number of cultural taboos – most specifically sex and death. Families sometimes feel they cannot even acknowledge that the person has died.

Homophobia: Many gay and bisexual men become alienated from their families. Some are rejected outright by their families. Gay people often move away from their families of origin and live far away at the time of their diagnosis and illness. Religious institutions can reject people at a time when the support of the religious institution is really needed.

Multiple loss: People who are dying from HIV/AIDS have often seen friends die and families often experience multiple losses when more than one child or grandchild has died from the illness.

Suicidal ideation: Suicidal ideation and attempted and completed suicides appear to be more common among the population struggling with AIDS.

Alcohol and substance abuse: There are significant problems with drug and alcohol use within the gay and bisexual male community. Those who have particular problems are at increased risk for relapse or increased use during the bereavement process in an attempt to anaesthetize the pain of grief.

Conclusion

This chapter has given a brief introduction to counselling and the steps that make up the counselling process, i.e. attending, listening, empathizing, questioning, probing, and summarizing. These skills are used in the pre-test and post-test counselling process, in the crisis intervention process, and in bereavement counselling. It is important for people involved in providing home-based care to ensure that community caregivers are given training in the skill of counselling. They also need ongoing support for this difficult part of their work. This can take the form of group supervision sessions where they can discuss their own emotional reactions and difficulties with the counselling task. It can also involve further training to sharpen skills.

References

Beuster, J. 1997. 'Psychopathy from a traditional S.A. perspective'. *UNISA Psychologia* 24 (2): 4–16.

Bodibe, R.C. and T. Sodi. 1997. 'Indigenous Healing'. In D. Foster, M. Freeman, and Y. Pillay (eds.) *Mental Health Policy Issues for South Africa*, pp. 181–92. Pinelands: Medical Association of Southern Africa.

Bowlby, J. 1969. *Attachment and Loss*, Vol. 1, 'Attachment'. London: Hogarth Press & The Institute of Psycho-analysis.

Bowlby, J. 1977. 'The making and breaking of affectional bonds'. *British Journal of Psychiatry* 130: 201–210 and 421–431.

Buhrman, M.V. 1986. *Living in Two Worlds.* Illinois, Chiron.

Egan, G. 1990. *The Skilled Helper: A Systematic Approach to Effective Helping,* 4th Edition. Los Angeles, CA: Brooks/Cole Publishing Company.

Gilliland, B.E. and R.K. James. (2001) *Crisis Intervention Strategies,* 4th Edition. Los Angeles, CA: Pacific Grove.

Hammond-Tooke, D. 1989. *Rituals & Medicines.* Johannesburg: A.D. Donker.

Kubler-Ross, E. 1989. *On Death and Dying.* London: Tavistock-Routledge.

Mbiti, J.S. 1969. *African Religions and Philosophy.* London: Heinemann.

Van Dyk, A. 2001. *HIV/AIDS Care and Counselling – A Multidisciplinary Approach,* 2nd Edition. Cape Town: Maskew-Miller Longman.

Whaley, S. and D.L. Wong. 1999. *Nursing Care of Infants and Children,* 6th Edition. Mosby: St. Louis.

Worden, J.W. 1991. *Grief Counselling and Grief Therapy,* 2nd Edition. London: Tavistock.

Recommended reading

Andrews, S. 2001. 'Informed consent and HIV'. *South African Journal of HIV Medicine* August: 10–12.

Bekker, L.G. 2002. 'HIV counselling'. *Southern African Journal of HIV Medicine* July: 30–1.

Frankl, V.E. 1991. *Man's Search for Meaning.* London: Hodder and Stoughton.

Helquist M., Dilley J.W., and C. Pies. 1989. *Face to Face – A Guide to AIDS Counselling.* San Francisco: AIDS Health Project, University of California.

Marcus C. and J. Knott. 2002. *Hospice Caregivers' Training Manual.* Johannesburg: Hospice Association of Witwatersrand, South Africa.

Oliviere D., Hargreaves R., and B. Monroe.1998. *Good Practices in Palliative Care – A Psychosocial Perspective.* Sydney: Ashgate Arena.

Poss, S. 1993. *Towards Death with Dignity: Caring for Dying People.* Boston: George Allen & Union.

Rogers, C. 1965. *Client-centred Therapy.* Boston: Houghton-Mifflin Company.

Running support groups for people with HIV/AIDS

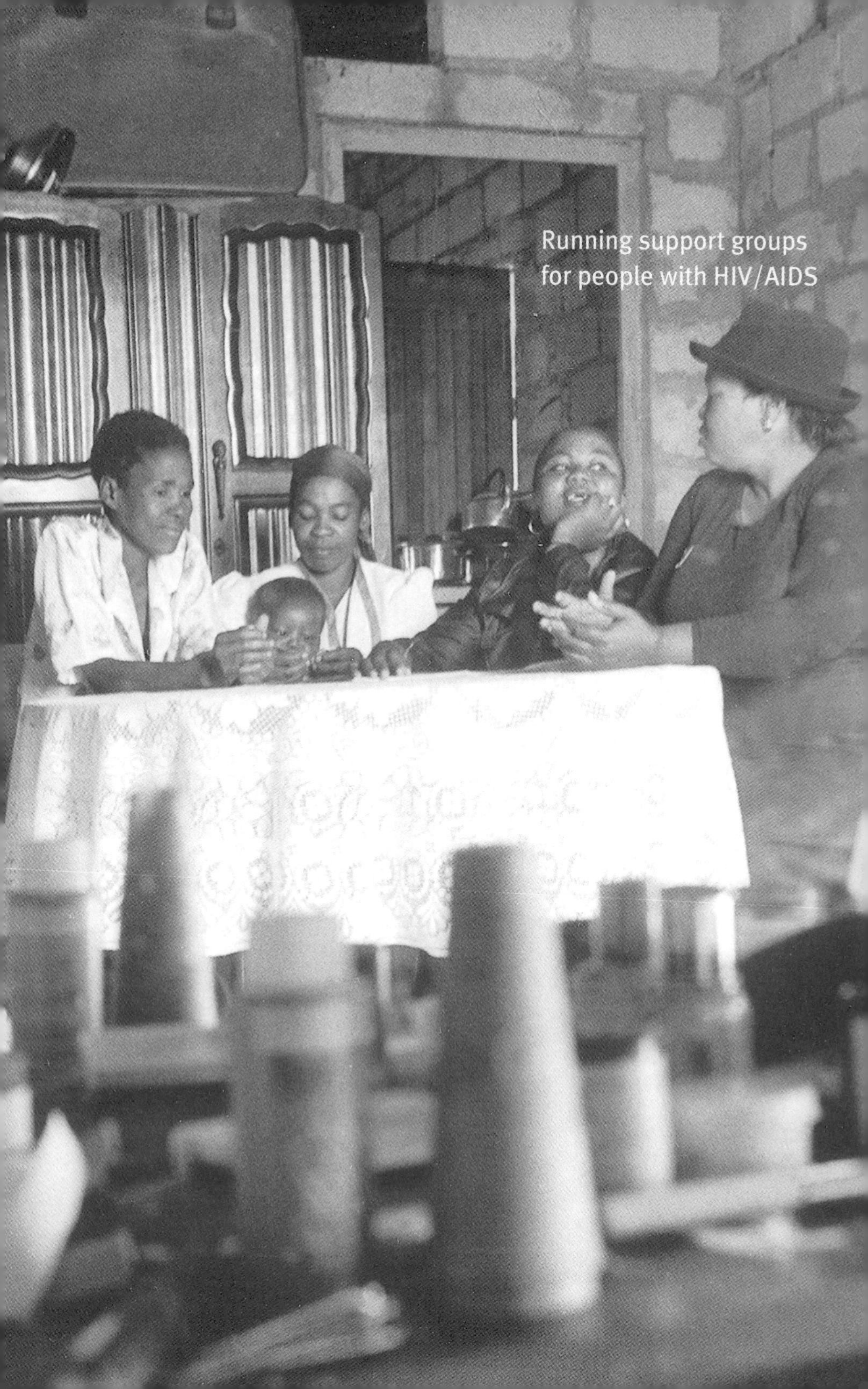

5 Running support groups for people with HIV/AIDS

Stefan Blom and Carey Bremridge

If there is one thing I feel I have learned from my adult life, lived inside an unreliable body, it is that care not cure will keep us floating in the ocean (Weingarten 2001, 124).

Introduction

A holistic continuum of HIV prevention and care structures is needed to prevent the stigmatization, discrimination, and trauma associated with HIV/AIDS. If there are no such supportive structures, discrimination against people with HIV infection can continue, and it might be inappropriate to offer voluntary counselling and testing (VCT) services. One support structure that can be considered, is group work that offers support to people infected with HIV and other diseases.

Support and self-help groups have been proposed as a key intervention for people living with illness. Support groups are described as structures where 'people meet on a regular basis to talk about their difficulties or simply to relax and enjoy each other's company' (van Dyk 2001, 251).

Informal structures such as family, friends, and neighbours are individuals or groups that care for the sick people they know out of a sense of love or duty. Or they are people, such as members of a church who give time to community service (UNAIDS 2002).

These structures often offer care and support to individuals in their own homes (community-based home care), but can also take on a group format. However, sometimes even these carers need additional support from outside the immediate circle. Formal structures of support are often offered by people from the professional sector. Community health workers, nurses, doctors, psychologists, traditional healers, social workers and HIV/AIDS counsellors can be considered formal support members. They are volunteers or are employed and receive training and ongoing supervision. They offer individual and/or group support services (See Figure 5.1). Support groups are usually initiated by a professional person within a formal structure (a counsellor, psychologist, nurse, social worker, etc.), but are mostly coordinated and maintained by one or more members of the group (community). Members of a community that share the same interest, illness, or problem (for example HIV or sexual abuse) might also meet spontaneously (for example at a talk, meeting, or health care facility) and in time form a more structured support group.

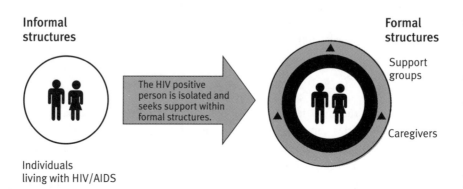

Figure 5.1 Individuals living with HIV/AIDS

What do people consider a supportive group?

Support defined in the context of support groups can be described as an environment and interaction that are safe, confidential, blame-free, informative, non-discriminating, respectful, understanding, and relevant (See Figure 5.2).

- *Safe:* A sense of trust in group members and leaders is essential. Members need to feel safe from possible discrimination and blame.
- *Confidential:* Group members also need to trust that personal information shared will not be discussed outside the boundaries of the group.
- *Free from discrimination and blame:* People join to experience the opposite of what group members' communities might offer – no blame for being HIV-positive. Any form of discrimination will break down the network of support.

- *Informative:* Group members also need appropriate information that might contribute to the experience of support.
- *Respectful:* Respectful behaviour (rather than words) contributes to trust and creates support.
- *Understanding:* A shared interest or life experience contributes to the feeling of being understood by group members, and this experience can be more valued than education or information (Swartz 1998). Group members can be considered to be 'experts' on their own lives, and this insider position on illness seems to be increasingly important for support (see for example, Epston 1998; Morgan 2000; Swartz 1998; UNAIDS 2002; van Dyk 2001; and White 1995, 2000).
- *Relevant:* Addressing the specific needs and expectations of each group member or group makes the group interaction relevant (Spirig 1998). Members should have an opportunity to break from the silence and isolation caused by a fear of discrimination. An HIV-positive person in a support group indicated that because he had a choice to disclose his status it was possible to let go of his secret (Browde and Nossel 2000). It is an opportunity to give and receive, to share, and to listen. Individuals witness others' experiences and are being witnessed by others – without being judged, blamed, or isolated. Support group members need to understand that talking is not enough. Actions, rather than words, create long-lasting networks of support.

Why do people join support groups?

The person living with HIV/AIDS might lose the support of family, friends, and community members through discrimination and stigma. Communities

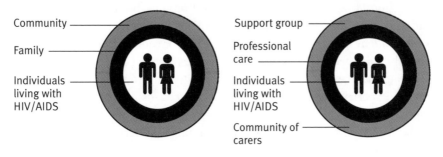

Figure 5.2 Support in the community

can convey a spoken or unspoken expectation of their members to withdraw themselves from those members carrying illnesses or disease – like HIV/AIDS (Weingarten 2001). In an attempt to break from the isolation, individuals may seek support and understanding elsewhere.

A key motivation for individuals to join support groups or self-help groups is that members seek a shared experience of a certain problem. This shared experience is often valued more highly than education and offers a built-in support system to group members (Swartz 1998; Yalom 1985). People join support groups to experience the following:

- Similar life experiences are shared and accepted.
- New perspectives or ways of thinking are learned.
- Members are motivated through the achievements of others.
- New and creative ways of managing problems are explored.
- An increase in trust and confidence in members is expressed through taking action against their life difficulties.
- Problem-solving skills are taught.
- Knowledge (information) and skills are offered.
- Relaxation and enjoyment are experienced in a safe and non-judgemental environment.
- Significant and gratifying interpersonal relationships are formed.
- Unique expectations and needs of group members are met.
- Hope is experienced and maintained.

Problems with support groups

Not all groups are described or experienced as supportive by their members. If the specific needs of a group member are not met, that member might experience the group as less supportive (Spirig 1998). For example, if an individual joins a group to learn more about treatment options, but only receives information on nutrition, that group member might experience the group as irrelevant or not as supportive. It is the group leader or coordinator's responsibility to see that the specific needs of group members are met.

Group members that have serious psychiatric disorders or drug addiction and are experiencing psychological trauma or crisis, or are mentally challenged, might not be suitable members for a support group (Yalom 1985). It also seems that when an individual is continuing to experience great difficulty in disclosing his or her status to anyone familiar (family or friends), individual counselling is recommended before group participation. These members need to address their individual needs and fears before sharing them with a group.

Any individual with specific needs that differ from the collective needs of a group might not benefit from a group experience, as the individual might not be able to contribute to others with responsibility, sensitivity, and care.

Why work in groups?

Group work can be described as an extension of individual support. Group work settings are considered a valuable tool in the breakdown of secrecy and isolation (Want and Williams 2000). Not only do groups provide support, but they also provide an audience of people who can witness and authenticate the process of change for every group member.

Group work is embraced as a valuable meeting place in which children and adults come together to talk and develop ideas about the nature, impact of, and ways of dealing with, problems in their lives (Want and Williams 2000).

The sharing of meaning and purpose can create emotional closeness and takes courage. But for this process of sharing to create closeness or cohesion, it is dependent on the listeners, on who listens and in what ways.

Instead of bearing the pain alone and believing that pain is inherently an individual and personal matter, the boundaries of support are expanded beyond our family to a community of caring persons (Weingarten 1999, 13–26).

The benefits of support groups, especially for terminally ill patients, have long been accepted into the mainstream thinking of medical care (Weingarten 1999). The AIDS Information Centre (AIC) in Uganda offers ongoing support groups to all clients, regardless of their HIV status. They found that:

On-going support helps HIV-positive members cope with infection and helps both HIV-positive and HIV-negative members adopt and maintain effective prevention behaviour (UNAIDS 2002, 18).

Members (of the so-called Post-Test Club) also help change social norms in support of HIV risk reduction.

Content

A closer look at different organizations' HIV/AIDS support group programmes reveals that a spectrum of emotional, psychological, and informa-

tional support is on offer (Spirig 1998; UNAIDS 2002). Broadly defined, these preventative and supportive services *focus* on:
- counselling
- nutrition
- medical care
- home visits
- practical and basic needs (like transport, employment, and food distribution)
- skills training
- job creation initiatives
- recreation
- HIV/AIDS education, and
- interpersonal and social support.

These services take on many forms within support groups, including:
- close interpersonal discussions
- guided/focus group discussions
- films and videos
- guest speakers
- drama group presentations
- questionnaires
- home visits, and
- meetings and seminars.

Creating or presenting boxes or books containing photos, stories, poems, and other mementoes of family and friends, can be an important tool or activity for the creation of support between support-group members and their families and friends (van Dyk 2001; see also Chapter 2). Often used as a way of dealing with grief, group members design books or boxes filled with information (stories, photos, etc.) that hold personal meaning and significance. As group members share their boxes or books with an audience of co-members or family members, a context for understanding and support is created.

Preparing leaders

Supporting the coordinators or group leaders of support groups is essential, but is often neglected. Assisting these caregivers with basic resources for the running of the group can be helpful, but more importantly, information on any of the following training topics seems to be useful:

Introductions

Different ways of making group members feel welcome, comfortable, and responsive towards others can be explored. Through sharing in a safe context, networks of support can be formed.

- *Contracting:* The importance of selecting basic guidelines of interaction for each group should not be neglected. Group members need to agree and stick to guidelines around meeting times, venues, duration of sessions, breaks, confidentiality, group expectations and needs, attendance, admittance of new members (or not), and other relevant matters that might influence the group session.
- *Group identity:* Based on the needs of group members, each group needs to decide what kind of group it would like. For example, group members can have closed (no new members allowed) or open groups (new members allowed); or a group can have a contracted lifespan (for example six sessions only) or an unlimited lifespan.
- *Basic education:* Group members that plan to maintain or support other groups need to consider different ways to present basic HIV/AIDS information in a manner that is realistic and, above all, practical and relevant.
- *Coping strategies:* Ways to access the coping abilities of group members and increase awareness in each person around their coping strategies or styles can be beneficial to group members.
- *Physical and medical care:* Exploring realistic ways to practise self-care in different forms like exercise, nutrition, and basic medical care is essential.
- *Group dynamics:* Finding a balance between the general patterns and constantly changing needs of individuals and the group as a whole is explored.
- *Closure:* The importance of ensuring the continuous safety of group members as they find the courage to share with others needs to be highlighted.

Getting started

While the importance and benefit of support-group work can easily be understood, the practice of establishing support group structures may at times prove problematic.

Group membership

Although PLHA (People living with HIV/AIDS) do share a common status, which may at times result in common or specific needs, remember that PLHA remain unique individuals from diverse populations. Support-group work for PLHA should never be understood as the cheap way to provide support for all those who cannot afford individual counselling. The golden rule around inclusion into support groups is simply that the individuals should want to be included. The individuals should feel that they will benefit from the experience of meeting, sharing, and learning with others who, like them, are HIV-positive. When selecting members for inclusion into HIV support groups, it is crucial that the specific need or interest of the individual be the guiding consideration. For some PLHA the need or interest might be to gain health or dietary information; for others the need might be to share interpersonal experiences. The success of the group will therefore always depend on the bringing together of PLHA who share a mutually expressed need. The specific need or focus of the group will also determine the ideal number of group members. Where the focus of the group is interpersonal discussion, the membership should be in the range of five to ten members, in order to afford each member adequate time to participate in the group discussion (Yalom 1985). The more members, the less time there will be for each member in the group.

Preparing support group members

It is important that the counsellor, nurse, or health care professional that refers the HIV-infected person to the support group should prepare each group member for the group experience. This would include discussing with the individual the specific needs that he or she is hoping will be addressed in the group situation, discussing the nature and process of the group, for example whether the group is a closed or open group, a discussion group, or a psycho-educational group, and highlighting the importance of confidentiality in the group setting. It is important that the individual has a clear understanding of the objective or focus of the group. In addition, it should be made clear that the group only provides a specific type of support and that the individual will still have access to individual counselling, medical assistance, information, and family support outside of the group setting. In this way, the focus of the group is well delineated and issues that are not appropriate for group discussion can be addressed in other settings.

Logistical requirements

Before a support group is established, certain logistical decisions need to be made. It is important that the venue for the group be equally accessible to all group members. In practice, difficulty in finding transport to and from the venue is often reported as an obstacle to attendance. Where necessary, transport might have to be arranged, but it is important that this is done without compromising the privacy and confidentiality of each group member. One should also avoid taking too much responsibility for group members. As stated earlier, it is essential that members should want to attend the group and make the necessary commitment to arrange transport to attend. In addition, it is important that group facilitators should not 'steal' the HIV-infected person's independence by continually 'over-care-taking'. The venue for the group must be a secure and safe place, which will regularly be available at the time of group sessions. 'Secure and safe' should also be understood as free from interruption or exposure to non-group members. This can prove a difficult task in practice, as clinic or hospital settings often have limited space and there are seldom group rooms available, which are out of the public eye. The time that group sessions are held is also important, as many members might not be able to attend during working hours. However, if the group meets after hours some group members might be afraid to explain their attendance of the group to family members or friends to whom they have not disclosed their status. Family commitments or safety in travelling home might once again be obstacles to attendance. The time of group meetings, frequency of group meetings, and the life span of the group will therefore have to be determined by the group members' needs. The duration of each session will depend on the focus of the group. It has been indicated that for full and equal participation of all group members in interpersonal discussion groups, group sessions should range from one to two hours (Yalom 1985).

Confidentiality

One of the most challenging tasks for effective HIV/AIDS support-group work is providing the guarantee of confidentiality for all group members. In many communities the stigma of HIV/AIDS still remains and discrimination against PLHA still occurs, despite legislation that clearly states that discrimination is unlawful. Given this context, the importance of confidentiality, and the implications should there be a breach in confidentiality, need to be emphasized each time the group meets. This is extremely important in small communities where group members are likely to see each other or each other's family members or friends outside of the group setting. In larger communities, it is common to use only the first names of group members. In addition, the group members should be given the choice as to whether process notes may be taken and where such notes will be kept. For those who have access to the Internet, many Internet chat rooms have been established as 'virtual support groups' for HIV-positive persons, but even on the world-wide web, one's anonymity is not always guaranteed. What is important to remember, however, is that, if appropriately selected, and given that each group member shares a common HIV-positive status, it is highly unlikely that any group member will disclose the identity or status of another group member. It is far more likely that each group member will share the common fear of discrimination, rejection, and pain of their fellow group members.

Group rules

Once the group has been established, it is important that the group members take ownership of the group and the time in group sessions. While it is common practice for health care professionals to initiate and facilitate support groups, it is essential that group members understand that the content of the session is dependent upon their need, interest, and participation. Group members should be encouraged by the facilitator to establish the context rules that will ensure that their mutually expressed need will be met during group sessions. Context rules would, for example, include basic rules (such as one person talks at a time) and more challenging issues (such as ensuring non-judgemental and respectful participation). If the group members have agreed that the support group will be a long-term group that will continue to meet until the group members agree to dissolve the group, the facilitator might also encourage the group members to run their own groups. By this it is meant that the facilitator would no longer lead the group and that the group would continue to meet together for as long as the group members had a common need to do so. The lifespan of a group should ideally be determined or governed by the mutual need to receive support. As long as there is a mutual need that is being met, group members should be encouraged to come together in a supportive and respectful context as frequently as is needed.

Conclusion

Despite these challenges and obstacles that can be met in trying to establish groups for HIV-positive persons, group work has been shown to offer caring, supporting, and empowering experiences for PLHA. Group work can also provide the necessary support and knowledge for family members or friends of PLHA or family and friends who feel isolated and fear the stigma of having lost a loved one to HIV/AIDS. In addition, support groups have been shown to be of great value to health care professionals working in the HIV/AIDS field.

References

Browde, P. and M. Nossel. 2000. 'Friendship and community in the age of HIV: a conference collection'. *Dulwich Centre Journal* 1&2: 53–61.

Epston, D. 1998. *'Catching Up' with David Epston: A Collection of Narrative Practice-based Papers Published Between 1991–1996.* Adelaide: Dulwich Centre Publications.

Morgan, A. 2000. *What is Narrative Therapy? An Easy to Read Introduction.* Adelaide: Dulwich Centre Publications.

Spirig, R. 1998. 'Support groups for people living with HIV/AIDS: a review of literature'. *Journal of the Association of Nurses AIDS Care* 9 (4): 43–55.

Swartz, L. 1998. *Culture and Mental Health – A Southern African View.* Cape Town: Oxford University Press.

UNAIDS. 2002. *Caring for Carers: Managing Stress in Those Who Care for HIV/AIDS.* Geneva: Joint United Nations Programme on HIV/AIDS.

Van Dyk, A. 2001. *HIV/AIDS Care and Counselling. A Multidisciplinary Approach.* Cape Town. Maskew Miller Longman.

Want, C. and P. Williams. 2000. 'Adventures in groupwork'. *Dulwich Centre Journal* 1&2: 11–17.

Weingarten, K. 1999. 'The politics of illness narratives: who listens, who tells and who cares? Narrative therapy and Community work: a conference collection'. *Dulwich Centre Journal* 1&2: 13–26.

Weingarten, K. 2001. *Making Sense of Illness Narratives: Braiding Theory, Practice and the Embodied Life: Working with the Stories of Woman's Lives.* Adelaide: Dulwich Centre Publications.

White, M. 1995. *Re-authoring Lives: Interviews and Essays.* Adelaide. Dulwich Centre Publications.

White, M. 2000. *Reflections on Narrative Practice: Interviews and Essays.* Adelaide. Dulwich Centre Publications.

Yalom, I.D. 1985. *The Theory and Practice of Group Psychotherapy.* New York: Basic Books.

Recommended reading

Andersen, T. 1987. 'The reflecting team: dialogue and metadialogue in clinical work'. *Family Process* 26 (3): 415–428.

Couzens, A. 2000. 'Reconciling the past, the present and the future. Narrative therapy and community work: a conference collection'. *Dulwich Centre Journal* 1&2: 6–8.

Sliep, R. 1996. 'Conversation with AIDS and CARE'. *Dulwich Centre Newsletter* 3:5–11.

Weingarten, K. 2000. 'Witnessing, wonder and hope'. *Family Process* 39 (4): 389–402.

Wingard, B. 2000. 'Hopefulness and pride. Narrative therapy and community work: a conference collection'. *Dulwich Centre Journal* 1&2: 5–6.

Dealing with the symptoms of AIDS

Dealing with the symptoms of AIDS

6

Liz Gwyther and Joan Marston

Introduction

Palliative care is the active total care of patients whose disease is no longer responsive to curative treatment. Effective management of HIV-positive patients requires vigilant assessment of symptoms and prompt intervention in managing opportunistic infections and controlling symptoms. Encouragement of healthy lifestyle and nutrition are also important. With the high incidence of HIV infection in lower socio-economic groups, assisted feeding and food supplements have become a significant factor in managing HIV infection. It is undeniable that the most effective palliative treatment for HIV/AIDS is antiretroviral therapy (ART); however, the absence of such drugs does not mean that nothing can be done.

Indicators of HIV/AIDS

There are a number of tests that give an indication of whether a person has HIV/AIDS and how the illness is progressing. These are summarized in Table 6.1. Not all of the tests will be available in clinics or public hospitals. However, this could be used as a guide and resources such as hospice associations might be able to assist with symptom control.

Other baseline investigations include:
- VDRL (Venereal Disease Research Laboratory) diagnosis of syphilis
- PAP test – there is a strong correlation between HIV and human papillomavirus, which is associated with an increased risk of carcinoma of the cervix
- sputum test for TB, and
- chest X-ray if the patient has fever, weight loss, cough, haemoptysis.

Table 6.1 Indicators of HIV/AIDS

Test	Result	Comment
HIV ELISA test	2 positive tests confirm diagnosis	Remember pre- and post-test counselling
CD4 count: Normal values 500–1 000 (Not available in most hospitals and clinics)	<350 symptomatic HIV infection <200 indicates susceptibility to infections <50 indicates very poor immune status	CD4 count fluctuates with current infections CD4 <50 evaluate interventions critically (e.g. decision whether or not to transfuse a patient with fatigue and weakness and low haemoglobin)
TLC (total lymphocyte count) from white cell count: Normal values (4–10 x 109) (Sometimes even this is not available)	<1.25 x 109 correlates with CD4 count of <200	Relatively inexpensive alternative to CD4 count
Viral load	Gives an indication of risk of progression to AIDS	For monitoring of patients on ART

Nutrition

HIV/AIDS has significant nutritional implications and consequences for the individual. There are three sets of factors that cause nutritional problems for PLHA, as outlined in Table 6.2. Early on in the illness, there may be few health problems, but a good diet during this time can boost the immune system and keep the person healthy for longer. Once the infections start, it is even more important to watch the diet, since the risk of depletion is greater, and it can lead to a dramatic collapse of the patient's defences. Studies have shown that opportunistic infections are more common in people with gross nutritional depletion (Department of Health 2001).

HIV/AIDS is an illness that affects the immune system. The immune system is made up of antibodies and cells (T- and B-cells) that attack invading germs. The T-cells directly attack the germs, while the B-cells manufacture the antibodies that assist in the fight. A high T-cell count indicates a healthy immune system (Department of Health 2001; Dube-Nxumalo 2002).

Table 6.2 Reasons for poor nutrition in PLHA

HIV/AIDS increases the need for food	HIV/AIDS lowers the intake of food	HIV/AIDS causes problems with food eaten
1. Because of the presence of the virus in the body, the immune system uses more energy to fight all the time 2. The person is worried, and this increases the need for food	1. General poor health decreases the appetite 2. Mouth and throat infections cause difficulties in eating 3. Medication affects eating 4. People are too tired to prepare meals 5. Lack of income limits food availability 6. Depression, worry, and anxiety decrease the appetite	1. Infections of the gut limit the ability of the body to absorb food 2. If the person has diarrhoea, nutrients are lost

Source: Department of Health 2001

Ensuring good nutrition starts early in the illness. While the person is still healthy, it is important to try to ensure a steady food supply. This may include planting one's own vegetable garden, and making sure that there are people who will maintain this when it becomes difficult for the PLHA. Another important early measure is to establish healthy eating habits, with a wide variety of foods, and a steady weight. If weight is lost, it should be replaced, if possible.

It is important to try to have all the food groups depicted in Figure 6.1 represented in a diet. Table 6.3 outlines some of the functions and sources of important foods.

Here are a few basic rules:

- Make starchy foods the basis of each meal. These foods, such as bread, porridge, pap, rice, potatoes, samp, millet, mealies, sorghum, and pasta are relatively cheap, and supply a lot of energy.
- Use unrefined, unprocessed foods. Unrefined means, for example, that bread should be whole-wheat, rice should be unpolished, maize meal should be stone-ground. This kind of food is much more nutritious than refined food.

Table 6.3 Functions of some important food groups

Type of benefit	Function	Sources
Proteins	Build the body and the immune system (T- and B-cells)	Beans, lentils, meat, fish
Vitamin C	Recovery from infections	Potatoes, cabbage, turnips, citrus, mangoes
Vitamin A	Keeps linings of gut, lungs, and skin healthy	Carrots, sweet potatoes, eggs, liver, pawpaw, apples
Vitamin B6	Maintains immune and nervous systems	Liver, beans, potatoes, banana
Vitamin B12	Production of T-cells	Milk, eggs, fish, meat, turnips, sunflower oil, mangoes
Vitamin E	Boost the immune system	Nuts
Zinc	Important for immune system	Meat, fish, whole-grain cereals, mealies, beans
Selenium	Activate the T-cells	Dairy
Iron	Builds blood supply	Whole-grain food, dairy, and protein-rich food Leafy green vegetables, whole-grain, meat, beans
Flavonoids	Prevent cancer and other diseases	Citrus fruit, apples, berries, carrots, cabbage, cauliflower
Phytosterols		Seafood, peas, seeds, whole-grain and many others
Water	Dissolve and excrete toxins	
Fats and sugar	Gives energy	Fatty meat, dairy, chocolate

Source: Dube-Nxumalo 2002

Figure 6.1 Food groups

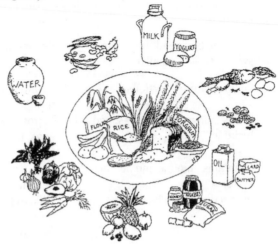

Source: Kennedy 2001, with permission

- Use fresh vegetables and fruit, since they provide more vitamins and minerals. What is grown locally is better than what has to be transported over long distances, since it loses many nutrients. Raw fruit and vegetables are also more nutritious than cooked or prepared vegetables.
- Add protein in the form of beans, lentils, peas, peanuts, soya, chicken, and fish. These are low in fat, but still give the necessary building material for the body. Local sources of protein such as mopani worms might also be added.
- Avoid too much fat, sugar, colouring, preservatives, and stimulants. If the person has thrush, sugar should be avoided, since it encourages thrush. If a person is losing weight, the fat and sugar intake should increase. Also avoid alcohol, since it damages the liver, and interferes with the absorption of nutrients.
- Use yoghurt, sour milk, and other dairy products frequently. Eggs are also highly nutritious (James 2000; Department of Health 2001).

Diet during diarrhoea

Avoid:
- all dairy products
- greasy, high-fat food

- high-fibre food
- apple juice
- sugar
- caffeine
- alcohol, and
- nicotine.

Eat more:
- white, starchy foods (oatmeal, potatoes, white rice, bananas, yams)
- guava juice
- non-caffeinated beverages
- salty things to replace salt lost, and
- vegetables and fruit.

Drink:
- soup, juice (especially apple, pear, peach, apricot, grape), water, black tea
- between meals rather than with meals, and
- remember that all carbonated cool drinks are high in caffeine.

Diet during constipation

Do: Eat regular meals to ensure bulk in the gut, drink lots of fluids, make sure you get regular exercise, and eat more roughage.

Avoid: Laxatives, which cause loss of water and salts. Don't delay going to the toilet when you feel the need to evacuate the bowel, since the urge will go away and the stools will get harder.

Low-cost diet

Good foods to include in a low-cost diet are: potatoes, peanut butter, baked beans, local in-season fruit and vegetables, concentrated fruit juices, and soya products.

Poor appetite

Do: Eat when you feel like it, and what you feel like eating. Eat smaller meals more frequently, take exercise, drink high energy drinks such as milk, maas, yoghurt, and mageu (a traditional sour-milk drink). Eat with your favourite people at your favourite place.

Too tired to prepare food

Do:

- Let others help you by preparing and bringing meals.
- Eat fruit and yoghurt, which gives energy but takes little effort to prepare.
- Leave food for a bed-ridden person in a cooler bag by the bed.
- Use canned or frozen food.

Diet for nausea

Do:

- Take smaller meals, or snacks.
- Try cold or chilled food.
- Eat dry toast, crackers, and cereal, which help to decrease nausea.
- Get somebody else to prepare the food.
- Avoid lying down immediately after eating.
- Replace lost fluids by taking soups, water, juice, and jelly.

The control of opportunistic infections

Tuberculosis is the commonest opportunistic infection in South Africa. Atypical presentation of TB is common in HIV, e.g. tuberculous lymphadenitis, serositis syndromes, and TB meningitis. The incidence of multi-drug resistant TB has increased with the HIV epidemic. Untreated TB causes sustained immunological stimulation, allowing HIV to replicate at a much faster rate and resulting in an increased viral load and a rapid fall in CD4 count.

HIV-infected patients who are infected with TB should be treated according to the national guidelines (Kennedy 2001). Direct treatment observation is important. Those patients who develop multi-drug resistant TB should be treated by specialized units according to specific protocols.

Management of opportunistic infections

HIV-infected patients who develop opportunistic infections should undergo appropriate investigations to establish an accurate diagnosis, and early anti-infective treatment should be initiated.

Table 6.2 Medication for opportunistic infections

Infection	Treatment
Community-acquired pneumonia	As per culture: (If available) Amoxycillin 250–500 mg 3 times a day for 5 days Cefuroxine 250–500 mg 2 times a day Clarithromycin 250–500 mg 2 times a day (Not on EDL code)
Pneumocystis carinii pneumonia (PCP)	Co-trimoxazole, e.g. 2 tablets, 3 times a day (1 tab/4 kg weight) for 3 weeks plus prednisone 40 mg 2 times a day for hypoxia
Giardiasis	Metronidazole 2 g daily for 3 days Metronidazole 400–800 mg 3 times a day for 5–10 days According to the South African National Formulary, the following regime is also applicable: Metronidazole 400 mg, 8 hourly for 5 days (8 hourly is 3 times a day).
Mycobacterium avium complex (MAC)	Clarithromycin 500 mg 12-hourly (if available) and ethambutol 15 mg per kg daily
Parasitic infestation	Albendazole 400 mg immediately (Not available in many hospitals)
Oesophageal candidiasis	Fluconazole 200 mg daily for 2 weeks
Cryptococcal meningitis	Amphotericin B IV, Fluconazole 400 mg immediately, 200 mg daily
Oral candidiasis	Nystatin solution, Amphotericin lozenges
Toxoplasmosis	Cotrimoxazole 4 twice a day for 4 weeks, 2 twice a day for 8 weeks

Source: Harley 1999

Prophylaxis

There are a number of opportunistic infections that are so common that in order to prevent them from occurring, treatment might be initiated before the patient has these infections. The following might be considered:

- prevention of PCP in patients with CD4 <200 by using co-trimoxazole two daily
- TB prophylaxis, but only once active TB has been eliminated (trials are continuing to assess the value of TB prophylaxis)
- life-long treatment for MAC, using clarithromycin 500 mg twice daily and ethambutol 15 mg/kg/daily (this is recommended, although it is not possible in the public sector)
- oesophageal candidiasis – fluconazole 150 mg daily for two weeks
- cryptococcal meningitis – fluconazole 200 mg daily, and
- toxoplasmosis – co-trimoxazole two twice daily for three months.

Nursing care

The nursing care of patients with opportunistic infections will be related to the symptoms, and whether there is a danger of cross-infection or not. Education of the family in dealing with infectious waste; infection control; and dealing with symptoms will be part of the nurse's responsibility. Special care should be taken in educating children who may be caring for parents or older siblings, in infection control.

Where possible, provide adequate resources, even if they are simple items such as plastic bags tied with rubber bands instead of gloves. Where the patient has a respiratory infection, they should be cared for in a separate room until treatment has rendered them non-infectious.

Where there is a possibility of the patient having fits, safety precautions must be implemented within the home, and basic first aid taught in dealing with this. Everyone in the household should receive education on how to position the patient on his or her side, with the airway extended to open it.

Dealing with pain

Effective pain control starts with accurate assessment of pain and frequent review of pain control. Remember that the concept of total pain encompasses physical pain, emotional pain, psychological pain, and spiritual pain. A patient with HIV may have more than one cause of physical pain. Assess quality of pain (description), radiation of pain, site of pain, duration and character of pain, and the effect of pain on the morale of the patient.

Common causes of pain in specific areas of the body in HIV/AIDS are:

- oropharyngeal pain: *Candida,* herpesviruses, cytomegalovirus (CMV), gingivitis, ulcers
- retrosternal pain: oesophageal candida, reflux oesophagitis, *Pneumocystis carinii* pneumonia
- headache: toxoplasmosis, cryptococcal meningitis, cerebral lymphoma; the headache of cryptococcal meningitis can be severe and intractable and may require serial tapping of 10–20 ml cerebrospinal fluid
- abdominal cramps: diarrhoea and infection, and
- perianal pain: herpes simplex, *Candida.*

Management of pain should follow the World Health Organization's guidelines (Evian 1993), i.e. by mouth, by the clock, and by the ladder.

- *By mouth:* Pain medication should be given orally at all times, since this assures best absorption, and avoids the complications of injections.
- *By the clock:* Pain medication should be given regularly, as prescribed, and not given only when the patient is complaining of pain.
- *By the ladder:* Pain medication should be increased in a step-by-step manner:

    Step one: Non-opioid ± adjuvant analgesic, e.g. paracetamol or aspirin
    Step two: A weak opioid ± adjuvant analgesic, e.g. codeine and aspirin (Codis) or codeine and paracetamol (Paracodol) ± non-opioid
    Step three: A strong opioid ± adjuvant analgesic, e.g. morphine ± non-opioid

Do

Morphine is the most commonly used strong opioid analgesic and should not be withheld from patients experiencing severe pain. Mist morphine must be administered four-hourly. The usual starting dose is 10–20 mg four-hourly and this dose is titrated upwards depending on the patient's analgesic requirements. There is no ceiling dose for morphine.

Morphine has a number of side-effects, such as temporary confusion, drowsiness, nausea, and/or vomiting and constipation. Tolerance occurs to morphine's side-effects, except constipation. It is therefore important to prescribe laxatives concomitantly with morphine. Myoclonus (twitching of muscles) may occur especially in the last few days of life, as morphine metabolites accumulate due to renal failure. (Treat myclonus with diazepam or lorazepam, rehydration, and a reduced dose of morphine.)

Morphine does *not* cause respiratory depression in therapeutic dosage and is useful in managing the sensation of dyspnoea. Pain is a physiological antagonist to respiratory depression.

Physiological addiction is not seen, but caution should be used when prescribing for patients with pre-existing addiction. Inflammatory mediators, which are produced in terminal illness, block kappa-receptors (which are the receptors responsible for the euphoric effect of recreational drugs). That is why addiction is not seen in palliative care use of morphine (Suzuki, et al. 2001).

Don't

Do not use pethidine! Pethidine is a partial opioid analgesic. It has a short half-life and is inappropriate for regular administration. It is also poorly absorbed orally. Repeated use results in a build up of toxic metabolites that cause convulsions.

Do

- Use adjuvant analgesics, such as non-steroidal anti-inflammatory drugs.
- Corticosteroids can be used if the pain is caused by inflammation and oedema. Corticosteroids are anti-inflammatory medications. Dexamethasone 8–16 mg daily as a starting dose is appropriate, reducing the dose to maintenance of 1–2 mg daily.
- Antidepressant medication can be used for neuropathic pain. Amitryptilline 25–75 mg at night.
- Anticonvulsant medication can be used for neuropathic pain. Carbemazepine 50–100 mg four times daily.
- Antispasmodics can be used for abdominal pain. Hyoscine 10–40 mg three times a day. (This is not available in oral form in most hospitals.)

Peripheral neuropathy

The causes of neuropathic pain are HIV, alcohol, vitamin B deficiency, and certain drugs.

Treatment options include:

- thiamine 100 mg daily
- pyridoxine (vitamin B6) 50 mg
- morphine – neuropathic pain is partially responsive to morphine
- amitriptyline 25–75 mg at night, or
- carbemazepine 50–100 mg four times daily.

If the above combination has not improved neuropathic pain, a further option is ketamine 100–200 mg once daily in a syringe driver. (This is not available in most hospitals.)

Nursing care of the patient in pain

Together with the medical treatment, certain nursing actions may assist with pain management. The nurse is usually the person who teaches the patient and family about pain management and the various drugs available. Nursing care for pain includes:

- accurate recording of the pain, its site, any medication given, and the reaction to pain medication or other therapy
- massaging the painful area gently
- applying warmth or cold to the affected area
- immobilizing and/or supporting a painful joint or area
- providing pain medication thirty minutes before carrying out a procedure that may be painful
- practising aromatherapy or reflexology
- offering music therapy or other forms of distractive therapy
- helping with the activities of living to reduce unnecessary movement
- massaging to reduce lymphoedema
- counselling and giving emotional support, and
- providing a soft, soothing diet when the patient has oral candidiasis.

Cough and/or dyspnoea

There may be many different causes of cough and dyspnoea in HIV/AIDS. Some of the commoner causes include sinusitis, PCP, Kaposi's sarcoma, TB, and pleural effusion.

Management of respiratory symptoms includes the following steps:

- Treat infections, e.g. with anti-tuberculous therapy.

- Provide PCP prophylaxis. All patients with a CD4 count <200 or a TLC <1.25 × 10⁹ should be using co-trimoxazole, one daily, to prevent PCP.
- Drain effusions.
- Give a bronchodilator for bronchospasm.
- Give physiotherapy.
- Administer hyoscine 10–40 mg three times a day to reduce respiratory secretions. (This may not be available in clinics.)
- Mist morphine (at a low dose) can be used for dyspnoea.
- Dexamethasone is useful for dyspnoea and hypoxia.

Nursing care

- The patient should sit upright when dyspnoeic or coughing. Assist the patient to find the most comfortable position that allows him or her to breathe as easily as possible, and then use cushions and pillows to support the patient in that position.
- Dyspnoea is very frightening and the patient may feel safer if the caregiver or nurse remains with him or her.
- Oxygen may be given, making use of a humidifier.
- Keep the patient in a clear space so that he or she does not feel closed in, if possible near an open window.
- Keep the area dust free.
- Prevent people from smoking in that room or area and take care that paraffin stoves do not release fumes into the area.
- Three drops of eucalyptus oil on a teaspoon of sugar may help to subdue the cough.
- Keep sputum in a covered container and dispose of it safely.
- Observe for signs of haemoptysis and report this immediately.

Gastro-intestinal symptoms

Diarrhoea

Important causes of diarrhoea in HIV-infected patients are *Salmonella, Giardia, Campylobacter, Clostridium difficile,* CMV, *Cryptosporidium, Mycosporidium,* and HIV diarrhoea. Accurate diagnosis requires laboratory analysis of stool samples and in some cases biopsy.

Treatment of diarrhoea involves an appropriate antibiotic or anti-protozoal. If a definitive diagnosis cannot be reached, a course of ciprofloxacin 250–500mg twice daily for three to five days may be prescribed or neomycin 1 g three times per day for three days. Ensure adequate hydration and nutrition. A lactose-free diet is advisable for seven to ten days.

Anti-diarrhoeals may improve comfort, e.g.:

- loperamide two immediately and one when necessary to a maximum of six daily (this might not be available in clinics), or
- codeine phosphate 30 mg six- to eight-hourly.

Nursing care

This includes maintaining a good fluid intake by giving frequent drinks of an oral rehydration fluid, either a commercially made product or a mixture of a litre of cool, boiled water, half a teaspoon of salt, and eight teaspoons of sugar.

The patient should be helped to keep clean after every stool and the anal area should be washed gently and protected from excoriation with a protective cream such as zinc ointment, or Vaseline. Diarrhoea may cause painful and bleeding haemorrhoids. If these bleed, a block of ice wrapped in a soft cloth can be put against the anus to control the bleeding and reduce the swelling.

For unpleasant odours that distress the patient, family, and visitors, a small bowl of vanilla essence or charcoal can be placed under the bed, to absorb the odours. A commercial air-freshener may also be used, or a bunch of lavender or another pleasant aromatic herb, near the bed.

Frequent sips of water or ice chips will help to control dryness of the mouth, together with a lip cream or Vaseline.

Constipation

If the patient is able to eat properly, constipation can be addressed by adding roughage to the diet in the form of fresh fruit and vegetables, stewed fruit, prune juice, grated beetroot, high-fibre cereals, and oats porridge. Extra fibre may be added to cereals, porridge, or soup. If adding extra fibre, the patient must be able to drink extra fluids.

Medications include stimulant Senokot, two to eight tablets at night, plus stool softener – liquid paraffin (1 tablespoon in orange juice) at night, or Lactulose. Many patients use home remedies such as Marula Jam and Black Forest Tea. Keep to the familiar remedy if it is effective for the patient.

Glycerine suppositories to soften the stool may be inserted rectally. Biscodyl suppositories may also be used to treat the constipation. If the patient has an impaction, soften the stool with a 100 ml warm olive oil instillation for an hour and then give a gentle warm water enema. Manual removal of faeces may be indicated to make the patient feel comfortable.

It is important that all patients using opioid analgesics should also be prescribed a stool softener and stimulation to prevent constipation.

Anorexia, nausea, vomiting

The most common causes of these distressing symptoms are *Candida,* malignancy, drugs, and constipation.

The management includes the following steps:

- Review the Candida treatment that the patient is receiving.
- Use the appropriate antiemetics – metoclopramide for gastro-intestinal-induced nausea, haloperidol for drug or anxiety-induced nausea, cyclizine for vestibular-induced nausea and nausea of raised intra-cranial pressure.
- Dexamethasone is used for managing raised intra-cranial pressure: 4–8 mg twice daily to start with, reducing the dose to a maintenance of 1–2 mg per day.
- Dietary advice can help greatly to address the problem. The appetite can be stimulated by giving small meals or snacks two to three hourly. Extra fluids and low-fat, unspiced food cause less nausea. Keep the mouth fresh with a mouthwash of 1 teaspoon salt/vinegar/lemon juice in 1 litre of water. Try small amounts of alcohol before meals, if not contraindicated. Avoid food with strong odours.
- Steroids may be used to stimulate appetite, e.g. dexamethasone 1–2 mg orally six-hourly.
- Give nutritional supplements like Ensure, Complan, PVM, and vitamin supplements.

Nursing care

- Prepare the food in small but appetizing portions, on a small plate.
- Sit patients upright while eating or drinking, and keep them in the upright position for 20–30 minutes afterwards.
- If patients need to lie down, ensure that they lie on their side with their head slightly raised, to protect against aspiration of vomitus.
- Keep a kidney dish or other container within reach of the patient.
- Give sips of cold water, or ice chips, hourly.

- Weak black tea, rooibos, or herbal tea may be tolerated well. Rooibos tea can also be an appetite stimulant.
- Chart the frequency and amount of vomiting, and teach the family to do this.
- Observe for signs of dehydration.

Pruritis and other skin conditions

The most common causes of skin problems in patients with HIV/AIDS are seborrhoeic dermatitis, papular urticaria, drug reactions, scabies, and folliculitis.

The management depends on the underlying condition:
- Folliculitis responds to flucloxacillin 250–500 mg six-hourly.
- Shingles responds to valaciclovir (not available in most hospitals) 1 g three times per day or aciclovir 800 mg five times a day for one week. Start within 72 hours. (For disseminated herpes give IV aciclovir.)
- Molluscum contagiosum responds to local treatment with liquid nitrogen (but this is not available in most hospitals).
- Sebborhoeic dermatitis responds to topical corticosteroids. Check for concurrent fungal infection.
- Papular urticaria may be caused by scabies and benzyl benzoate application should be applied initially. An antihistamine and aqueous cream may be beneficial, and topical steroids can be tried.
- Anti-scabies treatment – apply benzyl benzoate. Tetmosol soap lathered on and washed off the following day is also effective if the patient has scabies.

Nursing care

- Keep the skin clean by washing with a gentle soap and water. Add a spoon of aqueous cream to soften the water. Pat dry gently.
- Protect the skin by dressing the patient in clothing that covers the affected area.
- Dressings must be disposed of safely.
- Teach patients not to scratch the affected area, and to wash their hands before and after touching the affected area.
- Children may need to have mittens made for their hands from soft cloth to prevent them scratching.

Delirium and dementia

The confusion of delirium and dementia is very distressing for the patient and family. Zidovudine (AZT) is very effective in reversing AIDS dementia for a period of time.

Ensure a safe and, if possible, familiar environment for the patient. Take advantage of lucid intervals and explain the process to the patient and family. A calm, supportive familiar companion helps in the disorientation felt by the patient. Provide emotional support for the family.

Haloperidol can be used for agitation and anxiety. The recommended dose varies according to the patient's requirements, starting at 1.5 mg at night to 5–10 mg at night and 1.5–2.5 mg daily. Dexamethasone can be used if cerebral oedema is suspected.

Nursing care

- The safety of the patient may require that a bed be made up on the floor if he or she is very restless and inclined to climb out of bed.
- Soft music can be calming.
- Ensure that the patient gets enough food and fluids, and is kept clean and dry.
- Try to keep the environment quiet, without sudden loud noises that can startle the patient.

Other symptoms

Incontinence

Incontinence needs careful nursing care, rather than medication. Keep the patient clean and dry. Preserve the integrity of the skin with protective creams such as Vaseline or Fissan paste. Use adult disposable nappies if available, or large towelling nappies. Protect the bed with plastic sheeting. Incinerate disposable nappies. Support the patient and caretakers with the burden of this condition, emotionally and physically, and treat the unpleasant odours with charcoal or vanilla essence in the room. Where there is no other form of protection for the bedding, newspapers can be used.

Anxiety and insomnia

Anxiety and insomnia require psycho-social support and counselling in the first instance.

The following interventions may be useful:

- avoid alcohol and stimulants in the evening (suggest warm milk or herbal tea at night)
- relaxation techniques, such as aromatherapy, massage, and reflexology
- spiritual counselling, and
- medication, such as:
  - anxiolytics, e.g. diazepam 5 mg three times a day
  - alprazolam 0,25–1 mg three to four times a day
  - midazolam (useful as a subcutaneous medication in the syringe driver 5–15 mg daily), and
  - sedatives, e.g. oxazepam 10–15 mg at night.

Fatigue and weakness

It is important to diagnose specific conditions that might cause the fatigue. For instance, assess the patient's mental state, since depression may be a cause of fatigue and requires counselling and appropriate antidepressant medication.

- Check the full blood count and treat anaemia with iron and Vitamin B_6 supplements, as appropriate.
- Blood transfusion is indicated. If the haemoglobin goes below 7 g per cent, transfuse three to four units packed cells. The decision to re-transfuse depends on the patient's functional state and on the effect of previous transfusions. This decision needs to be individualized for each patient. However, a poor response to a previous transfusion, a CD4 count of <50 (TLC <75 × 10^9) in a bed-ridden patient would predispose to a decision not to transfuse again.
- Teaching patients to 'listen to their bodies' and to rest when tired, is essential.
- Adequate nutrition and nutritional supplements can also help, depending on the stage of the disease. Patients with poor nutritional status appear to do better with multivitamin supplements.
- Assistance with the daily activities of living, such as bathing, dressing, and feeding, and providing aids such as wheelchairs, walkers, and bath aids can be useful.
- Ensure a safe environment and supervision when a patient is in danger of falling.

- Promote independence for as long as possible by allowing the patient to take care of his- or herself with only the necessary assistance.
- Prevent pressure sores from developing once the patient is bedridden by regularly turning the patient, and by promoting good nutrition and hydration.
- Pressure sores are often difficult to cure, and frequently become infected. They may need hydrocolloid wound dressings where these are available. These are emotionally distressing for the patient and the family, who will need education on the care of pressure sores, and counselling. Where hydrocolloid dressings are not available, or not affordable, the sores must be kept clean and can be treated with a number of local remedies and available dressings. The dressings must be disposed of safely.
- High-energy drinks used by athletes and cyclists are pleasant and palatable, and may boost energy for short periods of time.
- Patients often need help with maintaining good oral hygiene, and hair and nail care.
- Even when the body is fatigued, the patient may enjoy mental stimulation such as having a book or story read to him or her, listening to music, watching television, or engaging in pleasant conversation.

Conclusion

The symptom control of patients with AIDS depends on combining good nursing care with prudent medical treatment. It is important to assess the patient's degree of immunosuppression (which correlates well with total lymphocyte count) and clinical condition. Care of the terminally ill involves a holistic approach, so evaluation of psychological state, social issues, and spiritual issues is also important. Palliative care is best carried out by an interdisciplinary team, so the patient's primary health care worker needs to be vigilant in identifying problems that could best be managed by another member of the team.

Effective and early diagnosis and management of opportunistic infections and physical symptoms is essential in order to achieve the best quality of life for the patient and family.

References

Department of Health. 2001. *South African national guidelines on nutrition for people living with TB, HIV/AIDS and other chronic debilitating conditions,* www.sahealthinfo.org/nutrition/sanational.htm (last accessed: 16 November 2002).

Dube-Nxumalo, M. 2002. 'HIV/AIDS and nutrition'. *Umbiko 3* (September): 8.

Evian, C. 1993. *Primary AIDS Care.* Cape Town: Jacana Education.

Harley, B. 1999. *HIV/AIDS Primary Care Clinical Guidelines, Cape Metropolitan Area.* Cape Town: City Health Department.

James, J.S. 2000. 'Nutrition and HIV infection: Experience in Zimbabwe – Interview with Lynde Francis'. In *AIDS Treatment News* 355, www.thebody.com/atn/355/interview.html (last accessed: 15 November 2002).

Kennedy, R.D. 2001. *South African National Guidelines on Nutrition for People Living with TB, HIV/AIDS and other Chronic Debilitating Conditions.* Department of Health, www.sahealthinfo.org/nutrition/sanational.htm (last accessed 10 March 2003).

Suzuki, T., Kishimoto, Y., Ozaki, S., and M. Narita. 2001. 'Mechanism of opioid dependence and interaction between opioid receptors'. *European Journal of Pain* 5 (Suppl A): 63–5.

Recommended reading

AIDS Nutrition Services Alliance (ANSA). 2002. '24 Living on a limited budget'. In *Nutrition fact sheets,* www.aidsnutrition.org/FactSheets/Main.aspx (last accessed: 15 November 2002).

Aids Nutrition Services Alliance (ANSA). 2002. '4 Treatment for Diarrhea' In *Nutrition fact sheets,* www.aidsnutrition.org/FactSheets/Main.aspx (last accessed: 15 November 2002).

Doyle, D. and N. Hanks. 1999. The *Oxford Textbook of Palliative Medicine,* 2nd Edition. Oxford: Oxford University Press.

Maartens, G. and L.G. Bekker. 2001. 'Deciding when to institute terminal care for AIDS patients – an evidence-based approach'. *South African Medical Journal* 91 (7): 559–60.

SA Hospice Association. 1998. *Guidelines to palliative care in HIV/AIDS.* Pinelands: Hospice Association of South Africa.

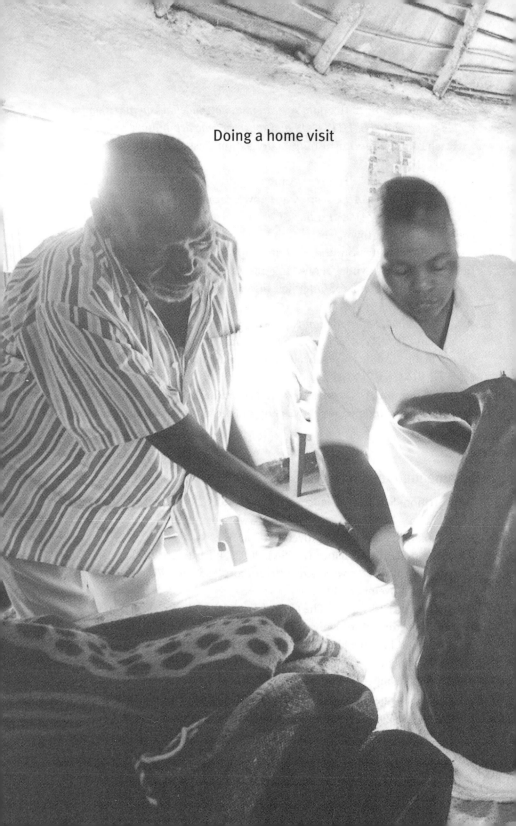

Doing a home visit

7 Doing a home visit

Joan Marston

Introduction

The home visit is central to the concept of home-based care. It enables the health care worker to make a realistic assessment of the PLHA and family's holistic needs, and provide care and support that is suited to the individual circumstances of each PLHA.

Within their own homes, PLHAs tend to be more open about their emotions, fears, and needs than they are in the strange environment of a hospital or clinic. Family dynamics are more easily observed and the educational and training needs of PLHAs and families assessed more effectively. While most PLHAs prefer to remain within their own homes, there are times when the home may not be a suitable venue for care, or when there may be no one to provide that care.

(For ease of expression 'family' will be used in the broader sense, to include relatives, and those caring for the PLHA within the home.)

The objectives of the home visit

The health care worker may visit the home for a variety of reasons:
- to introduce the health care worker to the PLHA and family within a familiar environment
- to explain to the PLHA and family the purpose of providing home-based care
- to make an holistic assessment of the PLHA and family
- to plan care and support, involving the PLHA and family in all stages of the planning
- to evaluate the educational and training needs of the PLHA and family, and to plan to meet those needs

- to evaluate the need for human, material, and social resources
- to identify both actual and potential problems, and to develop a realistic plan to alleviate these problems
- to assess whether or when the PLHA and/or family may need to be referred to other agencies
- to manage pain and other symptoms
- to identify children in distress (CINDI) and plan for their care and support
- to identify actual and potential bereavement issues
- to provide counselling for the PLHA and/or family and to help them come to terms with death and dying
- to ensure a safe environment for the PLHA and family, including control of infections
- to provide the best possible quality of life for the PLHA
- to assist with bereavement after the PLHA's death, and
- to empower PLHA and families to become as independent as possible in aspects of care and self-care.

The home-care team

The home-care team should be coordinated by a professional nurse assisted by trained community caregivers (CCGs) and other trained volunteers; with the support of the PLHA's doctor and other members of the interdisciplinary team, who will then be referred to as necessary for each individual PLHA. Other categories of nurses may also be involved in home care.

Before making home visits, all members of the team must receive appropriate training, including training in the principles of palliative care. All members of the team should have good communication and interpersonal skills, and the ability to empathize with others.

The professional nurse

Ideally, the professional nurse would be trained in palliative care and community nursing care. Psychiatric nursing, or training in counselling, would be an advantage.

The nurse should be able to carry out a thorough physical examination, and be able to identify psychological problems.

The professional nurse should ideally also carry out the first home visit and develop the PLHA's care plan, together with the PLHA and family.

When CCGs carry out the basic visits and day-to-day care, the nurse would still pay regular visits to the home to evaluate the progress of the PLHA and the effectiveness of care. The frequency of visits depends on the number of PLHA, the size of the area that is supervised, the needs of each PLHA, and the level of competence of the CCGs.

The professional nurse also mentors and supervises the CCGs and other nurses.

In most cases, the professional nurse would be the main channel of communication with the doctor and other members of the interdisciplinary team.

Community caregivers

As much of the basic care, support, and assessment of the PLHA and family are carried out by the CCGs, they must have a comprehensive theoretical and practical training. This is not only for the protection of the PLHA, but also for their own protection against infection, injury, and emotional burnout. The CCGs may be employed, or may be volunteers. The functions of the CCGs are discussed further in Chapter 3.

As they are usually members of the community they serve, the PLHA and families find them acceptable.

Volunteers

Volunteers come from a variety of backgrounds. They may be trained and experienced professionals, trained CCGs, family members, or compassionate members of communities who wish to reach out and help those in need.

No matter what their background, volunteers should not be sent to do home visits before they have a good basic training and understand the physical, spiritual, psycho-social, and emotional conditions they may encounter, and how to deal with these. They should also be evaluated on their suitability for involvement in this field. Volunteers would liaise regularly with the professional nurse in charge of the PLHA's care.

Often the volunteers involved in the care of a particular PLHA belong to the family, or are friends or neighbours. In some instances they may be children. The importance of training, supervision, and support for all categories of volunteer should never be neglected.

The PLHA

While it is usual to see the PLHA as the focus of the team, but not part of it, in home-based care the PLHA and the family take responsibility for the care most of the time. The PLHA is therefore the central and most important member of the home-care team and, wherever possible, must be involved in the planning and implementation of care and should be kept informed of any changes in the programme. The autonomy of the PLHA should always be protected and promoted by making PLHA part of the decision-making process.

Through self-care training the PLHA can be assisted to reduce the incidence of opportunistic infections. Even something as simple as good oral hygiene contributes to improved quality and length of life.

Everything possible must be done to meet the PLHA's need for information and training, and respect should be shown for their contribution to decision making and to the team. No procedures can be carried out without informed consent being given.

In the event of the PLHA being too sick, too young or, in any other way incapable of making decisions or giving consent, either the legal guardian or the next-of-kin may make these decisions.

Referring PLHA for a home visit

PLHA for the home-care programme may be referred from a variety of sources. Within most programmes, anyone may refer a PLHA – a doctor, nurse, social worker, clergyperson, family member, friend, or the PLHA his- or herself. It is usual to ensure that the person to be visited knows about the visit and consents to it. In the case of a child, the parent or guardian should agree. Where the PLHA is unable to give consent because of weakness or disability, the nearest relative should agree to the visit.

The PLHA has the right to refuse a visit.

It is advisable to contact the PLHA's own doctor and inform him or her of the first intended visit. This provides an opportunity to gain more information on the PLHA, and opens a channel of communication for the future.

The first home visit

The first home visit should, ideally, be carried out by a professional nurse. This may not always be possible, and a CCG may have to perform a preliminary assessment until the professional nurse can get to the PLHA.

This home visit should be carried out within seventy-two hours of the PLHA being referred to the programme.

The first home visit may be delayed because of a number of factors:

- The PLHA may live in an area that is difficult to reach because of distance, poor roads, bad weather, or unrest in that area.
- The home-care team may cover a large area and not be working in the PLHA's area at that time.
- The professional nurse may have a number of prior referrals or other essential visits to make.
- The PLHA may not give immediate consent to the visit.

Most delays could be minimized if there were trained and supervised CCGs living and working within each smaller community.

At least one to two hours should be set aside for the first home visit for the following reasons:

- This enables the nurse to meet the PLHA and family members and to inform them of the objectives of home-based care.
- The PLHA can be examined in a relaxed, unhurried manner, and rapport established between the PLHA, family, and nurse.
- The effectiveness of the PLHA's medication, and the need for further medication can be assessed.
- Pain and other symptoms can be diagnosed and treatment begun.
- Physical weakness and/or disabilities can be evaluated.
- A psycho-social evaluation can be carried out and plans made to access grants or other forms of social relief.
- Family dynamics can be observed along with the ability of the family/caretakers to care for the PLHA.
- The effect of the illness on any children made vulnerable by HIV/AIDS may be observed.
- Information can be obtained to begin with a spiritual assessment.
- Contact details of the PLHA, family members, doctor, clinic, employer, clergyperson, and any other relevant person, can be obtained.
- The nurse can begin to develop a care plan, together with the PLHA and family.
- A genogram can be completed to put the patient in the context of a relationship network.
- The need for information, education, and training in that home can be assessed.

- The PLHA's need for training in self-care can be evaluated.
- Information to assist with possible welfare grants can be obtained.
- The nurse can evaluate whether the PLHA needs any assistant devices such as a wheelchair or walking frame.
- The safety of the PLHA's environment, including the need for infection control measures, can be assessed.
- The need for any type of emergency intervention or admission to a care facility can be made.

The holistic assessment

Assessment of the PLHA and family should be holistic, i.e. physical, spiritual, psycho-social, and emotional issues should be taken into account.

The physical assessment

The nurse should have the knowledge and skill to carry out a thorough physical examination. Apart from noting physical symptoms and abnormalities, the PLHA's ability to carry out the activities of living will need to be assessed. Weakness brought on by the progress of the disease, actual physical disability, malnutrition, depression, and youth or advanced age can impair the PLHA's ability to carry out these activities.

The nurse will need to take a full and detailed history of the PLHA's physical symptoms and their treatment and list the medications that the PLHA is taking, as well as evaluating any possible drug interactions.

The effectiveness of each treatment also needs to be noted.

The nurse should examine the following for impaired function, infection, or disease:

- the cardio-vascular system – noting pulse rate and rhythm, shortness of breath, swelling of the ankles, or other signs of odoema
- the respiratory system – noting rate, rhythm, and type of respiration, signs of respiratory distress, cyanosis, signs of infection, history of tuberculosis or *Pneumosistis carinii* pneumomia
- the neurological system – including loss of vision or hearing, ataxia, muscle weakness, dementia, and peripheral nerve dysfunction
- the genito-urinary system – including sexually transmitted diseases and whether the PLHA is pregnant, breast-feeding, or planning to fall pregnant
- the condition of the skin – including signs of infection, Kaposi's sarcoma,

dehydration, and pressure sores

- the general nutritional state – signs of kwashiorkor, marasmus, cachexia, vitamin deficiency, weight loss; if possible, weigh and measure the PLHA
- the digestive system – dysphagia, anorexia, candidiasis, oral lesions, hairy leukoplakia, dental caries, and gingivitis may be present; a history of the incidence of diarrhoea should be taken
- lymph-node enlargement
- the ability to carry out the activities of living
- the PLHA's general hygiene
- the level of pain (this assessment may be carried out using a variety of instruments), and
- the stage of the disease.

A full description of the findings should be recorded. This is often done by means of a detailed form or forms, and may include a pain chart, and a picture of the front and back of the body. See Appendix C for an example of such a form.

Basic observations that should be taken include the temperature, pulse, respiration, and blood pressure. Weight and height may also be measured, but this is not always possible. Practical procedures may need to be carried out, such as bathing the PLHA or dressing a wound. Family members can be taught to perform simple procedures and may enjoy being involved in these aspects of care. Where there is no one in the home to assist with these procedures, the health care worker will have to plan visits to carry these out.

The supervision of DOTS may form part of the home visit.

Specimens of blood, sputum, stool, and urine may need to be collected during the visit. Care must be taken to store these correctly and safely.

The spiritual assessment

It is seldom possible to make a full spiritual assessment during the first visit, but details of membership of a religious group or church, and the name and contact details of the priest, pastor, imam, rabbi or other religious leader should be noted. These records should be made available to the interdisciplinary team, if this is acceptable to the PLHA.

The PLHA or family's reactions to being asked for these details will often give an indication of the role that religion plays in their lives, as will religious pictures or images that may be present.

The deeper spiritual issues such as their views on the meaning of life, illness, and suffering are usually only discussed once they know the health care worker better – if they are discussed at all. For some, this is a time of re-awakening of their awareness of religion and spirituality.

Emotions shown may include guilt at having 'sinned' and, therefore, being punished by God or a higher power; anger towards God for having caused or allowed the condition; bargaining with God (good behaviour in return for healing); or an acceptance of dying and a looking forward to an afterlife.

Whether or not the health care worker has the same views as the PLHA, he or she should accept and respect the importance of these beliefs in the PLHA's life. Respect must also be shown for different traditions and rituals. The health care worker should take time to discover the particular beliefs and rituals included in the different religions.

The psycho-social assessment

HIV and AIDS often lead to a number of psychological and social problems that may affect interpersonal relationships and cause tension within the home. The psycho-social assessment should include the PLHA as well as the family. Dementia may complicate the assessment of psychological reactions to the multiple losses and stresses experienced by the PLHA.

Psycho-social problems identified may include:

- denial of the infection or the extent of the disease
- guilt – including the guilt of having caused infection in others, such as a partner or child
- fear – of the unknown future, of death, of the reactions of others, of possible losses
- anger – towards God, towards the person who infected them, towards others who are healthy
- depression and thoughts of suicide
- altered sleep patterns
- uncertainty, anxiety
- coping with multiple losses and the fear of these losses, such as the loss of friends, health, independence, job and income
- coping with changed body image
- coping with changes in sexuality and sexual practices
- financial concerns
- changes in relationships

- concerns about pregnancy, possible pregnancies, babies, and children
- bereavement, and
- concern by parents for their children and other family members once they have died.

Counselling may be needed and may be adequately carried out by the health care worker, or may require referral to a psychiatrist, social worker, or psychologist. Often what is needed is an empathic and patient listener, to allow the PLHA and family to make their own decisions and develop their own coping skills. It is often sufficient for PLHA to be able to express their emotions, and have someone listen to, and respect their feelings. The health care worker may also find that simply providing the correct information may allay fears. In many cases just the knowledge that someone will be available to help them is sufficient to reassure PLHA and their families.

Where children are involved, issues such as whether the child is attending school or not, who supports the child emotionally, and the extent of the child's vulnerability will all need to be assessed.

Assistance with obtaining available grants and pensions is a long process and steps should be set in motion to obtain these from the first visit, especially for those living in extreme poverty, and where vulnerable children are involved.

Completing the first visit

The health care worker will need to discuss further visits by herself or another member of the team and leave contact details for the PLHA and family. Plans should be made to address training needs and any urgent training, such as in infection control, should be started. Educational pamphlets in the PLHA's home language, if possible, may be helpful. Emergency social relief will require immediate action, as will attention to the needs of vulnerable children.

Ongoing visits

With each visit, a holistic assessment will have to be carried out to evaluate:
- the progress of the disease
- the effectiveness of training
- the effectiveness of counselling
- the effectiveness of pain and symptom management and medication

- the ongoing safety of the environment
- the impact on family members with a special evaluation of children
- the ability of the PLHA to carry out the activities of living
- special needs to be met
- necessary referrals to be made to other agencies or to other members of the interdisciplinary team
- nutritional status and nutritional needs
- hydration
- the impact of the disease on the PLHA
- new symptoms, infections, or diseases, and
- the impact of the disease on the PLHA's sexuality.

The CCG should know when to refer the PLHA to the professional nurse, doctor, or social worker. Apart from these referrals, the professional nurse should also see the PLHA on a regular basis.

During regular visits, rapport is built up between the health care worker and the PLHA and family and this facilitates open communication.

The health care worker should tactfully discover whether the PLHA has a valid will, and, when this is not so, try to persuade him or her to make one.

Education of the family

Wherever possible, the family should be included in the education and training within the home. Children who care for adults need extra training and supervision and, ideally, adult support.

Education on the prevention of HIV/AIDS can be given effectively within the home. The use and making of simple home remedies may be taught. These are often cost-effective and acceptable. In many cases, the family teaches the health care worker about these home remedies.

The home-care kit

Table 7.1 gives an example of a basic home-care kit that can be used by the nurse or CCG. Medications may be added to the nurse's kit.

For CCGs and nurses who do their home visits on foot, a small backpack might be a useful way to carry the kit. For people using vehicles a small suitcase might be useful, since it can also be used as a table to set out equipment while working.

Table 7.1 Home-care kit

Equipment for CCGs
- clinical thermometer (oral)
- scissors
- nail clippers
- notebook
- home visit reporting forms
- hand soap
- plastic soap box/container
- torch (pen-light)
- batteries (pen-light)
- umbrella
- disposable Carlton paper/ paper towel
- PVC washable apron
- household bleach
- toilet paper
- plastic straws (bending)
- linen savers
- disposable latex gloves (size 71/2)
- napkins (adult)
- napkins (child)
- urosheaths
- urine bags
- sanitary pads
- syringe 10cc (feeding)
- newspaper
- black bags and plastic bags for waste and protection

Resource bank equipment
- bowl (for dressings)
- kidney dish
- foam mattress
- raincoat
- condoms
- bedpan
- urinal
- crutches
- wheelchair
- information brochures or sheets

Equipment for dressings
- spray bottle
- salt
- wooden spatulas
- gauze swabs
- sterile dressing packs
- gauze bandage 5 cm
- gauze bandage 10 cm
- micropore

Medication and nutritional support
- calamine lotion
- Vaseline
- aqueous cream
- betadine ointment
- gentian violet
- nystatin solution
- salt
- bicarbonate of soda
- rehydration solution
- cough mixture
- Valoid
- paracetamol tablets (500 mg)
- paracetamol syrup
- ferrous sulphate and folic acid tabs
- vitamin B Co tabs
- ascorbic acid tabs
- multivitamin syrup/tabs
- Ensure
- Morvite
- anti-diarrhoeal medication, such as Loperamide
- vinegar

Recording visits

Complete and accurate records should be kept of each visit. All records should be confidential and should be kept in a safe place.

The health care worker normally keeps records, but in some areas PLHA keep their own records. If the PLHA is taking special medication, e.g. for pain management, a medication chart should be left for the PLHA or family to complete.

Where PLHA have not disclosed their HIV status to the family, it is unwise to leave records in the home.

Special issues in home care

Quality of life

One of the aims of good palliative home-based care is the achievement of the best possible quality of life for the PLHA. Quality of life differs from person to person, but studies have shown some common factors:

- Quality of life is that which the PLHA identifies as such. This is a highly individual experience and may not be that which the health care worker identifies as quality of life. Ask PLHA what is needed for their lives to have quality. The answers are often unexpected.
- Quality of life depends on the presence of others – those whom the PLHA cares about, and those who care for the PLHA. The actual physical presence may not always be possible, but communication can be facilitated through telephone calls, letters, tape recordings, videos, and e-mail. Photographs of loved ones can be displayed where the PLHA can see them.
- Quality of life is achieved by attaining one's goals. Allow PLHA to identify their own goals and then set about creatively helping them to achieve them. A trip to Paris may be out of the question, but a Parisian evening, with a special meal, a sip of champagne, candles, French music, and a few red roses can create the atmosphere. Birthdays and special anniversaries can be celebrated early.
- Quality of life is related to maintaining hope. As the disease progresses, the focus of hope may change, and the PLHA may need help in changing the focus, but it should never be taken away.
- For some, simply providing shelter, nourishment, warmth, pain and symptom management, respect, and companionship may be all that is required to provide an acceptable quality of life. The therapeutic presence of the health care worker often provides comfort and security.

Ethical issues

Dealing with ethical issues during the home-care visit can, at times, be diffi-cult. Issues include the following:

- *Confidentiality:* PLHA may not wish their HIV status to be disclosed to their families or those caring for them. The health care worker should encourage PLHA to disclose, but respect any wish not to. Issues of infection control must, however, be dealt with for the safety of those caring within the home.

  The health care worker must maintain confidentiality at all times, and this includes keeping records where they cannot be read by others. Disclosure to anyone can only be done with the PLHA's consent, preferably also when knowledge of his or her HIV status is necessary for adequate care to be given.

- *PLHA autonomy:* The PLHA has the right to agree or disagree with pro-posed treatment. Providing the PLHA or guardian and family with detailed information allows them to make an informed choice.

- *Euthanasia:* Either the PLHA or the family may discuss the possibility of euthanasia with the health care worker. While this is illegal in South Africa, the concerns behind the request must be identified and discussed. Many fears can be addressed by good palliative care and counselling. Where there is a possibility of suicide, emergency psychiatric help is called for, and the PLHA should not be left unattended until the crisis is past.

- *Abortion:* An HIV-positive pregnant woman may wish to discuss the issue of abortion during the home visit. The health care worker cannot allow personal values to influence the PLHA's decision, but should give all the facts related to keeping the baby or procuring a legal abortion. Where a decision is made to obtain an abortion, the PLHA should be assisted to get the necessary counselling and should be provided with support.

Health promotion

The home visit is an ideal time to promote a healthy lifestyle, especially as the health care worker can evaluate the barriers to this within the home. Training can be given on good nutrition using the food that is available to the PLHA and family, within their financial resources. Assistance with developing a food garden, or advice on keeping chickens may help to promote good nutrition.

Training in hygiene and infection control promotes a clean and healthy environment for all in the home. The maintenance of good oral hygiene is important, and this can be achieved using a weak salt or vinegar and water solution, and a soft cloth.

The importance of adequate rest, fresh air, and gentle exercise where this is applicable can be discussed at each visit. With increasing weakness the PLHA may need to be reassured that it is important to rest, and not to feel guilty about this. Referral to the community occupational therapist where one is available may assist the PLHA to conserve energy and adapt to increasing weakness. Assistive devices such as wheelchairs, walking frames, toilet extensions or backrests may be required, and it may be necessary to plan for help with the daily activities of living.

The family or care giver within the home will need training to cope with these. The health care worker should be aware of the many 'teachable moments' that occur during the home visit and should use them effectively.

Sexuality and sex education

Within the privacy of the home, the PLHA often feels safe enough to discuss very personal issues. Sexuality may be affected by changed body image, physical changes, disease progression, and increasing weakness. Relationships may be affected because of this, and the PLHA and partner unable to discuss the issue or deal with it.

During a home visit the health care worker may need to facilitate discussion, or encourage PLHA to express their feelings on this subject.

Where PLHA are sexually active, issues of safer sex should be discussed as early as possible, and, when consent is given, sexual partners should be involved as well.

Caring for the dying at home

Most PLHA wish to be at home until they die. Where there is someone who can care for them adequately, with home visits by the professional nurses and CCGs for support, this remains the ideal.

However, there is often no one suitable to care for them at home, and then the home-based care team can be faced with a dilemma, as hospitals are reluctant to admit them at that stage. The CCGs may have to stay with the PLHA or make use of neighbours, other family members, or perhaps people from the PLHA's church, for full-time care. This situation should be planned for from the time of referral to the programme.

The home visits should become more frequent at this time for the following reasons:

- Care given by untrained caregivers at this time can be dangerous for them, as they will usually be dealing with infected body fluids, and have an inadequate knowledge of infection control.
- Pain and symptom management are essential for the PLHA's comfort and the family's peace of mind.
- The PLHA and family will require additional support at this time, to deal with the emotions associated with loss, and the fear of the unknown that is to be faced.
- All involved have to be prepared for the death. The health care worker should note the name and contact details of the chosen undertaker, and ensure that those caring for the PLHA know who to call. During the home visits, the family can be gently informed of the signs of impending death, and prepared for the care of the body once the PLHA has died.

Information should also be shared with all involved. Children and teenagers should not be excluded from the discussions, and should be kept informed of the PLHA's condition, using simple words.

Respect must be given to religious and cultural practices, as well as to the wishes of the PLHA and the family. When the PLHA has many visitors who tire him or her out, it is quite acceptable for the health care worker to limit visitors, or limit the length of the visit, with the PLHA's consent.

When death occurs at home

It is not always necessary, or possible, for the health care worker to be present at the time of death. Her or his work is to prepare the family to cope with the practical issues surrounding the death, such as calling the undertakers, and straightening the body.

A simple pamphlet, in the language of the family, can be provided. When death occurs, intense emotion can make people forget what they have been told, and having the information written down can help considerably.

A home visit should be made as soon as possible after the health care worker has received news of the death. When making this visit, time must be given for listening, observing emotions, determining whether people are coping with their grief, and answering any questions that the family may have. Assistance with funeral arrangements may be required. The health care worker is often asked to speak at the funeral, and the content of this speech can be discussed during the home visit.

Bereavement visits

At least one bereavement visit should be made to the family, usually within two weeks of the death. Where there is a bereavement programme, families can be informed of this and referred to the bereavement team. Each bereavement situation will be different, and different approaches to helping families deal with grief can be used.

When there are signs of complicated grieving, and where children are involved, more than one visit should be made, and individuals referred for professional help where necessary.

Staff and volunteer support

Working in the field of palliative care and support can be both physically and emotionally exhausting. Adequate annual leave and time off should be given. The person visiting the PLHA should have access to a support programme.

Working within a team, with regular supervision and mentoring (and regular support meetings), is usually effective, but the health care worker carrying out home visits should also have access to individual counselling.

Conclusion

Because of the extent of HIV and AIDS in communities, home-based care has become an essential aspect of the continuum of care.

Where trained health care workers provide this, visiting the PLHA on a regular basis and having access both to resources and to the members of an interdisciplinary team, a high quality of care can be provided cost-effectively.

Recommended reading

Doyle, D., Hanks, G., and N. Macdonald. 1995. *Oxford Textbook of Palliative Medicine*. Oxford: Oxford University Press.

Evian, C. 2000. *Primary AIDS Care,* 3rd Edition. Houghton: Jacana Education.

Hospice Association of South Africa. 1998. *Standards of Palliative Care.* Cape Town: Hospice Association of South Africa.

Ingleton, C. 1999. 'The view of patients and carers on one palliative care service'. *International Journal of Palliative Nursing* 5 (4): 187–95.

McDermott, R. 2000. *Palliative Care: A Shared Experience.* London, Ontario: Parkwood Hospital.

Sembhi, K. 1995. 'Palliative care in developing countries: Luxury or necessity'. *International Journal of Palliative Nursing* 1 (1): 48–52.

Uys, L. and J. Marston. 1998. *Palliative Care Standards.* Pretoria: Department of Health.

Infection prevention and control aspects in home-based health care

8 | Infection prevention and control aspects in home-based health care

Laura Ziady

Introduction

Infection control is a primary responsibility of all health care workers, whether they work in hospitals, in-patient clinics, or the home-based health care setting.

PLHA cared for at home often have the benefit of being in an area of low infection risk, as they are generally used to the micro-organisms in their own environment, and to those of their family members and regular caregivers. PLHA are usually more relaxed and less confused in their own environment and may feel that they have a measure of control over their lives. This will improve their inherent immunity, as they do not have the stress of being in a strange environment.

A negative aspect of home-based care is that the patient or PLHA is often immune-compromised for some reason, such as living with a life-limiting disease, or they may need hospital care that exposes them to infections. Hospitals may discharge patients suffering from communicable nosocomial infections (infections acquired in the hospital), the symptoms of which may only appear when the person reaches home. They can then transmit such infections to caregivers or family members. Limited resources, insufficient home-based care assistance, and a lack of equipment may make care more difficult, but much can be done with determination and initiative.

From the caregiver's side, an occupationally acquired infection (being infected by the patient while working) may cause temporary or even permanent disability and disease, affecting the caregiver as well as his or her family. A patient with a transmissible infection will need to take more thorough prevention measures than another whose condition is not contagious. For instance, a patient suffering from TB must adjust his or her way of coughing and disposing of coughed-up sputum. A standard programme teaching infection prevention and control will lead to a decrease in exposure to infection and an improvement in the knowledge and skill of the caregiver.

This chapter deals with strategies, infection prevention and control priorities, and methods for risk reduction, taking into account the patient and the service provider's economic, social, and home circumstances. Common infection control principles will be described, with some examples of their application. The goal is to guide home-based caregivers and service providers in the development of practical and innovative infection control programmes based on the patient's individual needs and resources. The rewards of a well-designed programme should be measurable in terms of improved care and lowered health care costs.

Word clarification

Readers may find many unfamiliar words in this chapter. These words are explained here.

Antimicrobial: A chemical agent used to combat infectious micro-organisms. The best example is antibiotics, a type of medication that is active against bacteria.

Antiseptic: A disinfectant that can be used on living skin and delicate surfaces as it will not damage the surface if used correctly.

Aseptic technique: A technique that ensures the absence of as many infectious micro-organisms as possible. Aseptic techniques are usually used when performing procedures with sterile instruments and equipment.

Diarrhoeal infection: An infection of the intestinal tract, usually following intake of infectious micro-organisms that leads to diarrhoea.

Infection prevention and control measures: Specific procedures and knowledge used to prevent the development or spread of infections among patients, staff members, caregivers, family members, visitors, and the environment.

Nosocomial infection: A hospital/clinic-acquired infection that developed later than forty eight hours after the patient was admitted to the hospital without any signs or symptoms of it, and is directly linked to hospital care.

Occupational acquired infection: An infection acquired while at work during normal or routine patient care tasks, without any sign or symptom thereof being present during the period before the work was done or contact was made with a patient.

Service provider: A private, para-statal, welfare, or non-governmental organization rendering a service to patients in their own homes or in an in-patient unit, by way of lay or trained health care staff.

Spores: A method of ensuring the micro-organism's continued existence when living conditions become hostile, e.g. drying or starvation. Example: A bacteria's genetic material is encased in a capsule, with loss of any non-essential protein and structures. In this format, the genetic material can survive for long periods until conditions become more conducive to proliferation, and germination then takes place.

Susceptible person: A person who can contract a disease because of a lack of resistance, e.g. against infectious micro-organisms.

Tincture: An antiseptic or disinfectant solution with alcohol as base.

Topical antiseptic agent: Antiseptics (disinfectants compatible with living tissue) that are applied to the skin's surface, e.g. hand disinfectant rubs that usually contain an emollient, and alcohol (and sometimes disinfectant).

Transmissible infection: An infection that can be spread from one person to another or from one surface to another through contact, droplet transfer, or airborne means.

Waste: Household – Waste that contains no potential or definite infectious ingredients, e.g. disposable paper, plastic, metal bottle caps, or kitchen refuse. It can be disposed of in a municipal landfill.

Medical – Waste that contains disposable items that have been in contact with a patient's blood or body fluids, e.g. wound dressings, paper tissues, incontinence nappies. This should be incinerated or buried.

Sharps – Disposable glass ampoules, vials or bottles; lancets; blood glucose pricks; scalpel blades that have been in contact with blood or body fluids, as well as any other items that can potentially break, abrade, cut, or damage a waste handler's skin or tissues. This should be incinerated or buried deeply.

Coordinating infection prevention and control activities

Providers of home-based care should try to ensure that family caregivers and community caregivers (CCGs), as well as patients are maximally protected against infection. To do this, they should develop a systematic infection control programme in the home-based care service.

The following process will assist in this task.

1. Assessing specific infection risks in home-based care settings is the first step in improving the quality of care. A standard assessment will help in devel-

oping realistic, prioritized objectives, defining the most practical procedure for each identified need, and incorporating methods to monitor results as time passes.

2. Develop a general, written infection control policy that outlines appropriate standardized measures for preventing or controlling infection for all CCGs and families. Criteria for selecting procedures for standardization include:

   • The procedures that hold the greatest infection risk for patients or caregivers should get the highest priority for standardizing. For example, protecting the caregiver from exposure to the body fluids of a patient with a blood-borne condition, such as infection with HIV, is as important as protecting the patient from external sources of infection.

   • Economic considerations and limited resources. Continuous provision of supplies such as plastic aprons, gloves, antiseptic soap and disinfectants, and treatments such as specific antimicrobials and topical antiseptic agents, combined with the need for special nutrition for the patient, and even the caregiver's need to use public transport, represent a substantial drain on available resources, whether for a service provider or an individual patient. Modern health care equipment and conveniences are often missing in poorer home care settings. Substitutes may be needed for items such as plastic protective sheets, bath basins, supportive devices, cushions, and other equipment. Imagination and creativity can produce many items for personal care and other procedures.

3. Educate and inform caregivers beforehand regarding:

   • all the possible infection control and prevention principles and procedures that they can use as the need arises in practice when caring for a patient

   • the use of standard precautions for general protection against exposure to infectious micro-organisms, and

   • sharing information such as the infectious status of a patient and which infection control measures can effectively be employed against the specific type of exposure.

Applying principles, such as the use of gloves to protect the carer's hands from contact with blood or body fluids during procedures is subject to adjustment according to individual patient circumstances. For example: In principle, blood and body fluids are always considered to be infectious, and caregivers are taught to use gloves to protect their hands from this type of contamination. If the patient or service provider cannot afford to buy the appropriate gloves, plastic shopping bags can be used to protect the hands.

4. Post-exposure management of occupational exposure is necessary where caregivers have been exposed to blood or body fluids, or have been injured in some manner. A standardized plan must be in place for incidents when a caregiver has been exposed to HIV, hepatitis B or C, TB, or any other contagious or transmissible disease. People who have suffered pricks, cuts, or abrasions of the skin or mucosa with sharp items used for patient care ('sharps injuries'); or splashes of blood or body fluid in the eyes or on nonintact skin or mucosa, should be informed about what to do.

Specific infection control and prevention strategies

Standard and special precautions

The Centres for Disease Control and Prevention (CDC) have identified certain standard, universal measures that will protect all patients and all caregivers from exposure to infection. These include scientifically sound basic practices and barrier precautions intended to reduce the risk of mutual exposure to micro-organisms, irrespective of whether the patient has a diagnosed infection or not. In a home-based care setting, these guidelines still apply, though they may need to be adjusted to individual circumstances.

Standard infection control precautions include handling all blood and body fluids as if contagious until proven otherwise, as well as using care practices that minimize the possibility of blood or body fluid contact.

At present the accepted practice is that all caregivers should implement standard precautions for all the patients they work with, while additional transmission-based precautions should be implemented for those patients with confirmed or suspected infections. For example:

- Precautions against infections that are airborne are appropriate for patients with confirmed or suspected pulmonary or laryngeal TB or multi-drug resistant TB. These patients are usually accommodated in a single room in a hospital or at home.
- Precautions against infections that are transmitted by droplets are primarily meant for patients with childhood respiratory transmissible diseases

such as mumps and chickenpox. The patient is usually accommodated in a single room in the hospital or separate from other susceptible persons in the home. People who are immune to the disease may come into contact or be accommodated in a single room with the patient, as long as they are not immune-compromised. Isolation of infected patients in separate accommodation has long been an accepted but controversial practice, and may be problematic in the home.

- Precautions against infections that are transmitted through contact are utilized for patients infected with diarrhoea, vomiting, skin conditions, blood-borne conditions such as HIV, or who have conditions where blood or body fluids may leak from intact skin, wounds, or broken skin areas and transmit infection.

Isolation precautions in home-based care settings consist mainly of:
- washing hands and hand disinfection
- using protective clothing and barriers
- keeping the environment very clean (environmental hygiene)
- cleaning, disinfecting, and sterilizing equipment, and
- maintaining a high level of personal hygiene for both the patient and the caregiver.

Physical isolation in the sense of separating a dying or very ill patient from his or her supporting family and friends is a decision that should not be lightly made. Protecting an immune-suppressed patient through strict isolation from all persons who might carry infectious micro-organisms may lengthen his or her life, but reduce its quality.

Hand washing and hand disinfection

This is the basis of all infection control practices. Both the caregiver and the patient should wash their hands whenever they are likely to have been soiled and before beginning any care procedures. Washing with running lukewarm water and enough soap to foam for the duration of the wash ensures that most transient micro-organisms are loosened and rinsed off the skin. Of those organisms left on the skin, at least 80 per cent will be removed through vigorous friction when wiping the hands, preferably on a paper towel that can be discarded afterwards.

Hands should always be washed, even if gloves have been worn. Not all gloves are 100 per cent impermeable and some may have pinprick areas that can leak.

Hands should always be washed when:

- visibly soiled
- if something known to be contaminated is touched
- before and after using the toilet
- before and after touching mucous membranes, non-intact skin, or moist body substances
- before meals
- before performing invasive procedures where the skin of the patient will be punctured, e.g. doing a blood glucose test, and
- when caring for patients known to be suffering from acute or chronic infections.

Ordinary hand washing with toilet or liquid soap should be done for at least thirty seconds, while scrubbing for any sterile care procedure such as wound care should be done with an antiseptic soap and should take a minimum of two minutes. If no antiseptic soap is available, ordinary soap and water must be used and the hands washed twice, the last wash lasting two minutes.

Antiseptic hand washing soap should preferably contain one of the following:

- 2–4 per cent chlorhexidine gluconate (best option)
- 70 per cent ethyl alcohol and 70–90 per cent isopropyl alcohol
- 2–3.5 per cent iodophors, or
- 1.5–3.5 per cent chloroxylenol.

Always use soap and water to remove blood or other organic materials from hands and surfaces. Avoid using basins filled with antiseptics or water to wash hands in as they are quickly contaminated and the stagnant water then becomes a source of micro-bacterial growth.

Soap for hand washing must be clean. Large bars of cracked, soiled soap lying in little pools of stagnant, dirty water are unacceptable. The topping up of partially empty containers of liquid soap is also a dangerous practice.

After washing, hands should be dried on either disposable paper or a clean, regularly laundered cloth towel.

When soap and running water are not available or the hands are not visibly soiled, waterless disinfectant rubs are suitable substitutes. This applies to the patient's hands as well. Waterless hand rubs must contain effective concentrations of antiseptics to check slight contamination. (Refer to Table 8.1) Spray bottles containing water and a fresh solution of either vinegar or bleach are relatively easy to transport for hand hygiene.

Where no running water is available at all, transport water in a container with a screw cap that can be poured by another person or hung up and tipped when necessary. The patient may need to conserve what water he or she has

Table 8.1 Hand hygiene procedures

Procedure	Product	Substitute
Hand washing	Soap Running water	A fresh solution of soap and water, and clean rinsing water in separate spray bottles are useful in areas where no running water is available
		Do not keep water in a container for longer than 24 hours as algae and bacteria will start growing in it
		Waterless hand disinfectant
Hand disinfection	Commercial products containing a mixture of antiseptics, alcohol, water, and emollients	1 part chlorine (household bleach) in 9 parts boiled, cooled water in a spray bottle. Change daily to a fresh solution as too much of the chlorine will evaporate within 24 hours to be an effective disinfectant
		1 part spirit vinegar in 9 parts boiled, cooled water in a spray bottle, mixed daily
		Wiping hands with a commercial 70% isopropyl alcohol wipe (not commonly recommended as this can severely dry out the hands)
		Wiping hands with a commercial wipe used for babies' bottoms (expensive)

available for drinking and cooking, and the caregiver should not use this for hand washing if possible.

Barrier prevention and control measures

The principle and aim of using infection control barriers is to keep moist body substances such as blood and body fluid off the skin and clothing of caregivers and patients. Examples of barrier precautions include:

- Double bagging highly contagious waste (such as the paper tissues used by a patient suffering from drug-resistant TB) or heavily soiled equipment and linen in a plastic inner 'dirty' bag and an outer 'clean' bag when handling items that are contaminated with blood, or when transporting contagious waste in a private vehicle to a disposal site. Double bagging contagious waste can protect the community in which a patient lives from exposure to infection in areas where sanitary waste removal is absent or uncontrolled.
- Protection of clothing is important to limit exposure of the caregiver to infectious micro-organisms but also to protect the susceptible patient from organisms that may be transmitted from the caregiver to the patient. Examples of protective clothing are listed in Table 8.2.

Environmental hygiene

Cleanliness is the first step in infection control and prevention. A high level of household hygiene is all that is required in the home-based patient care setting.

Cleaning entails the removal of all visible dust, organic matter (e.g. sputum, faeces, or blood), and things that do not belong (e.g. soiled plates, urinals, and linen), as well as a sufficient number of micro-organisms to reduce the risk of infection for all who have contact with the object or surface. Usually, if the environment looks clean, it is clean enough for good patient care at home. All good hygiene measures will directly and indirectly contribute to infection prevention and control.

All items handled frequently by the patient and caregiver(s), including articles soiled with blood or body fluids by the patient, should be washed and kept clean or disinfected immediately, or regularly enough that transmission of micro-organisms is unlikely to occur. The environment may harbour infectious micro-organisms (e.g. the bacteria that cause TB or diarrhoea). Good

Table 8.2 Protective clothing and measures

Area to be protected	Measure	Substitute
Hands	Medical gloves	Re-usable kitchen/garden gloves Plastic bags
Body	Impermeable surgical gown	Thin plastic raincoat Plastic refuse bag cut open for the head and arms
	Plastic apron	Rubberized overalls
Face (mouth and airways)	Mask Face shield	Head-scarf or large handkerchief over mouth and nose
Hair/head	Paper or cloth cap	Shower cap Head scarf/large handkerchief Plastic bag
Eyes	Mask with splash guard Visor Protective spectacles Goggles Face shield	Gardening goggles Welding spectacles Perspex face shield (e.g. used for soldering or welding)
Feet	Paper/plastic overshoes	Recycled plastic shopping bags anchored with sticky-tape or string
Environment	Plastic bags Paper for wrapping	Recycled plastic shopping bags Recycled newspaper

environmental hygiene includes keeping the patient's surroundings clean and tidy, ensuring that laundry (bed-linen and clothing) is done regularly so that the patient's skin can be kept comfortable, clean, and dry, and that meals are prepared, stored, and served in a hygienic manner.

Organizing patient care and housekeeping responsibilities is important. Careful planning is necessary, especially where there is no one else to help with tasks. Sometimes caregivers are required to do housekeeping tasks for the patients they are looking after. Where possible, the trained caregiver should not do any general housekeeping her- or himself, but should keep an eye on what is done in the home. Diplomatic guidance of household members to assist and to learn, and correct shortcomings in hygiene and cleanliness is always part of home-based care giving.

If there is no other choice, compulsory housekeeping tasks should be done after primary patient care has been completed, e.g. making patients comfortable or feeding them.

Table 8.3 gives examples of housekeeping tasks in the patient's direct environment.

Table 8.3 Household cleaning measures

Activity	Product/procedure used	Substitute/procedure used
Dusting	Commercial dusting product(s)	1 Part liquid detergent/machine washing detergent in 1 000 parts warm clean water – just dampen the duster in the solution to break the electrical charge that keeps dust clinging to surfaces
	Clean duster	Clean recycled cloth
Laundry/ washing soap	Laundry detergent	Washing machine detergent powder
	Surface cleaner	Grated toilet soap/scraps of toilet paper
	Dishwashing detergent	Carbolic bar soap
	Dedicated dish-/washcloth	Clean recycled cloth
	Hot water	Hot water
Damp mopping machine	Dampen the mop with clean water or a weak solution of the product used for washing the floor. Preferable to sweeping with a broom that only disturbs the dust	Dampen the mop with clean water or 1 part liquid detergent/washing soap powder in 1 000 parts warm clean water – just dip the mop or a clean recycled cloth in the solution and dry out. Preferable to sweeping with a broom which only disturbs the dust
	Rinse mop between rooms/when soiled, in clean water	Rinse mop/mop cloth between rooms/when soiled, in clean water
	Wash mop with soap and water and allow to dry after use	Wash out mop/mop cloth with soap and water and allow to dry after use

Table 8.3 *continued*

Wipe up fluid spills immediately	Use paper towels to wipe up spills (household spills or those of human origin). Place in a plastic bag afterwards and throw away Disinfect a spill of human origin by either covering it with paper towels soaked in a chlorine-based disinfectant, or pouring a disinfectant solution on it, leaving it to stand for at least 10 minutes before mopping it up and washing the area with soap and water	Use crumpled newspaper to wipe spills (household spills or of human origin). Discard into a plastic bag afterwards and throw away Wash spills of human origin with a cloth and soapy water. Disinfect a spill of human origin by either covering it with paper towels soaked in vinegar or by pouring a solution of 1 part vinegar in 9 parts boiled, cooled water (1:9 solution) over it and leaving it to stand for at least 10 minutes before mopping it up and washing the area with soap and water
	Allow surface to air-dry	Allow surface to air-dry
Cleaning kitchen and dry bathroom	Commercial disinfectant detergents/cleaners	Wash the environment with liquid detergent with warm water and air-
	Clean surface with dish-/washcloth sponge	Disinfect with 1:9 solution of chlorine (household bleach) in water or a 1:9 solution of vinegar in water
		Clean recycled cloth
Disposal of household waste	Seal in plastic refuse bags daily	Seal in recycled plastic shopping bags or wrap in old newspaper daily
	Put out for collection by the municipal sanitation department according to municipal regulations	Take to the local refuse landfill or burn at home

Table 8.3 *continued*

Activity	Product/Procedure used	Substitute/Procedure used
Waste disposal: • medical waste • 'sharps' • infectious liquid waste	Place 'sharps' in a sealed impermeable/waterproof container Seal medical waste in double plastic refuse bags Put both containers out for collection by the health care service provider/municipal sanitation department (check with Environmental Health Office of the local council). Incinerate or bury the containers in a deep, covered hole Infectious liquid waste can be flushed down a toilet bowl into a sanitary sewer	Place sharps in a rigid container/ double cardboard box placed out of reach Seal waste in recycled plastic shopping bags or wrap in old newspaper Incinerate both types of containers in a hole in the back yard daily. It will not be completely destroyed but will be un-recoverable. Cover with soil after cooling or bury deeply to prevent animal scavenging; or chemically disinfect with a chlorine-based product (cover with a solution delivering 1 000 ppm free chlorine) for 20 minutes before burial Avoid open piles of solid waste, or dumping waste in rivers, lakes, or areas where leaching can pollute water sources
Cleaning medical equipment	Clean, disinfect and store as prescribed in the manufacturer's guidelines or by the service provider's infection control policy	Clean, disinfect, and store as prescribed by the manufacturer's guidelines or the service provider's infection control policy
Cleaning cleaning equipment	Wash in warm soapy water, rinse in clean water and dry as far as possible in the sunlight Store dry Where a patient has a communicable disease that contaminates the environment, such as pulmonary TB in a patient with a productive cough, it may be necessary to use separate cleaning equipment for that area to prevent contamination of another area	Wash in warm soapy water, rinse in clean water and dry as far as possible in the sunlight

Disinfection and sterilization

Disinfection and sterilization are actually two points on the continuum of cleanliness.

Disinfection is a process that eliminates many or all growing micro-organisms on inanimate objects (not people, animals, or plants), excluding viruses and bacterial spores. Disinfection processes, including pasteurization, boiling, and chemical soaking, should kill all micro-organisms (excluding bacterial spores) within exposure times of less than thirty minutes after a load has attained the correct temperature.

There is a difference between 'disinfectants', and 'antiseptics,' which are used on living tissue. Disinfectants will damage living tissue because of their chemical properties, and products labelled 'disinfectants' must never be used instead of 'antiseptics' on living tissue.

Disinfection is always a two-step action, starting with cleaning/washing the interior and exterior surfaces of an object followed by disinfection with an appropriate chemical agent. An item cannot be properly disinfected if it hasn't been cleaned, because disinfectants are diluted, neutralized, or even de-activated by contamination or soiling (e.g. with organic residue), as well as the addition of more water or other chemical compounds (e.g. soap).

Disassemble instruments and equipment before cleaning and disinfection. Jointed or very intricate instruments that cannot be disassembled must be cleaned well and disinfected in an appropriate manner for the maximum period specified by the manufacturer of the instrument. The process is usually accomplished by soaking in chemical agents or by heat processes (boiling, pasteurization or baking, or exposure to dry heat).

The prerequisites for disinfection by boiling and pasteurization include that:

- only drinkable or boiled water, or water chlorinated to 0.1 per cent, is used
- all items must be clean or washed and rinsed beforehand
- items should always be completely submerged in the heated water
- air must be removed from hollow instruments or tubes during submerging
- no new item must be added to the load that has already begun to pasteurize or boil
- a disinfected item is removed from the container in which the procedure was done with clean washed hands or clean tongs or forceps, without contaminating it, before it is allowed to air-dry on a clean surface

- only dry items are considered adequately disinfected as the process continues during the drying stage, and
- clean water must be used for every new cycle of disinfection.

The disinfection time starts as soon as the coldest part of the load has reached the required temperature and is the actual period during which disinfection takes place. (This is called the holding or standing time.)

Table 8.4 Disinfection methods

Disinfection process	Contact time/ Holding time	Method
Boiling	100°C = 5–20 minutes 5 minutes is usually sufficient time for single items. Longer times are necessary at high altitudes, for overcrowded containers, and for complex, jointed instruments	Boil only items that are completely heat resistant at a temperature of 100°C. Boil in a clean, covered pot on the stove, a hot-plate, submerged in water in a microwave oven, or in a kettle over a fire. Boil gently as a rolling boil bounces items around, lowers the water level quickly and uses extra fuel. Using a pressure cooker speeds up the process. Air-dry on a clean surface, or dry items with a dedicated clean towel before storage or use *Advantages:* A reasonably cheap and reliable disinfection method *Disadvantages:* Time consuming and can be expensive. Devices with lumens or channels must be totally submerged and filled with water for the minimum holding time.

Table 8.4 continued

Disinfection process	Contact time/ Holding time	Method
Pasteurization	65 °C = 10 minutes 70 °C = 5 minutes 80 °C = 1 minute 90 °C = 1 second	Pasteurize only heat resistant items that can stand temperatures of 65–90 °C. The warmer the water the quicker the process and the less time needed. Pasteurize in a clean, covered pot or other heat-resistant container. The water can be heated in a container on the stove, over a fire or in a microwave oven, before the cleaned items are added, heated up, and the holding time starts, or the hot water can be poured over the cleaned items. The temperature must be higher than required, to allow for the cooling effect in both cases. Air-dry on a clean surface, or dry with a dedicated clean towel before storage or use *Advantages:* A cheap and reliable method *Disadvantages:* Time consuming and an be expensive. Devices with lumens or channels must be totally submerged and filled with water for the minimum holding time
Dry heat (baking)	160 °C = 60 minutes 180 °C = 30 minutes	Use only for completely heat resistant items, organic material, or linen as dry heat may cause discoloration and heat distortion. Dry heat penetrates surfaces less effectively

Table 8.4 continued

Disinfection process	Contact time/ Holding time	Method
		than steam or moist heat, and longer holding times are required. If possible, pre-heat the item at the same time as the oven, in a clean, closed container and then bake for the required holding time. Cool before use or handling *Advantages:* A cheap and reasonably reliable method *Disadvantages:* Time consuming, can be expensive and dangerous (exploding containers). Not a good choice for hollow devices or those items that have small lumens or channels, as dry heat cannot penetrate the hollows
Chemical disinfection (soaking, mopping, or wiping inanimate objects)	± 10 minutes–10 hours, following the manufacturer's guidelines	High-level disinfection is achieved when clean items are submerged in a fresh solution of disinfectant such as the aldehydes (8% formalin or 2% activated glutaraldehyde that will sterilize clean surfaces within 6–10 hours of continuous contact) or alcohols (isopropyl alcohol and methylated spirits) Mid-level disinfection is obtained with chemical agents such as the alcohols, halogens (including 0.5% household chlorine bleach, 1000 ppm free chlorine and povidon iodine), phenols (carbolic acid or Dettol®),

Table 8.4 continued

Disinfection process	Contact time/ Holding time	Method
		and acetic acid (e.g. spirit vinegar) that can destroy some growing bacteria, most viruses and fungi, excluding bacterial spores, within 20 minutes Low-level disinfection is provided with chemicals that can inhibit or destroy most growing bacteria, some viruses and fungi after 10 minutes. Example: Alcohols, halogens (Milton® or Domestos®), 0.5% chlorine solution in household bleach, quartenary ammonia compounds (Savlon®), and acetic acid (e.g. spirit vinegar) *Advantages:* Some chemicals are more readily available and cheaper than others are and can be used by most caregivers *Disadvantages:* Not all the above agents are as effective as traditional disinfectants, but will serve the purpose if used as directed in the home. All chemicals are deactivated/ neutralized to differing levels by contact with foreign material. Chemicals may leave a residue on the items being disinfected; be corrosive; give off noxious fumes and cause chemical burns if not washed off surfaces that come into contact with skin or mucosa;

Table 8.4 continued

Disinfection process	Contact time/ Holding time	Method
		and can be unreliable if used incorrectly as contaminated chemicals can become a source of infection themselves Devices that have lumens or channels must be submerged and filled with disinfectant for the minimum contact time. Micro-organisms can build up a resistance to disinfectants if they are used incorrectly. Chemical disinfection can be very expensive
Steam sterilization	*In a boiler/pot:* 100 °C = 20 minutes *In a pressure cooker:* 121 °C = 15minutes 126 °C = 10minutes 134 °C = 3minutes	A sterilization process destroys all micro-organisms, leaving surfaces free of all contamination. Sterility is only necessary when the item being processed will be penetrating a sterile body part such as the patient's blood circulation or tissues, e.g. during care of a deep wound. In home-based care, a high level of cleanliness or disinfection rather than total sterility is usually acceptable. Steam sterilization may be done in a home setting by suspending a washed item/instrument in a strainer over water boiling in a clean covered steam pot or pressure cooker. Sterilization will take place when steam condenses on the item for a period of time

Table 8.4 continued

Disinfection process	Contact time/ Holding time	Method
		Advantages: Reasonably cheap. Reliable if done correctly *Disadvantages:* Only applicable to heat-resistant solid objects. For all else, chemical sterilization must be used. Steam does not penetrate dry or waterless materials such as oils, grease, or powders. Can be dangerous (causing fumes/burns/ explosion of incorrectly handled containers)
Decontamination/disinfection of non-living surfaces/devices soiled with blood, or body fluids containing fresh blood (wiping/soaking)	Exposure time to the disinfectant: 1–10 minutes	1. Wipe contamination on solid surfaces with a paper towel or clean cloth 2. Wash with soapy water and a clean cloth, rinse and dry with the cloth 3. Wipe down with diluted chlorine (1: 9 water solution) or a commercial chemical disinfectant Washing surfaces with soap and water is cheaper and quicker than disinfection, preferably working with gloves. If no gloves are available, or if the surface is porous or the con- tamination is known to be highly contagious, soaking may be indicated If instruments or items cannot be washed immediately and must wait for a while before re-processing, they can be soaked in water containing bicarbonate of soda to keep

Table 8.4 continued

Disinfection process	Contact time/ Holding time	Method
		blood or body fluids from staining or hardening
		Rinsing contaminated linen in cold salt water before laundering in warm soapy water is preferable and cheaper than soaking it in a disinfectant solution
		If soaking of linen or clothing is required after heavy contamination with blood or body fluid, use a 0.5% chlorine solution for no longer than 10 minutes to prevent disintegration of material fibres/cloth. Wash, rinse and partially dry good quality re-usable kitchen or gardening gloves before completely submerging them in a disinfectant solution for 20 minutes for procedures such as wound care. Medical latex/rubber gloves tend to become sticky and useless after long exposure to harsh disinfectants
		Re-usable gloves to protect health-care givers from contact with blood or body fluids can be washed on the outside with soap and warm water (while wearing them), rinsed and hung up to dry
		Powdering the inside with a little talcum powder or starch makes them easier to put on again

Table 8.4 continued

Disinfection process	Contact time/ Holding time	Method
		Needles and syringes used for injections should not be reprocessed HIV and viral hepatitis have been transmitted by improperly processed syringes and needles in the past Syringes (and wide bore needles) used for drawing up baby feeds or medication should be disassembled, washed with soapy water, reassembled, the syringe filled with soapy water and ejected through the needle, before rinsing in clean water, followed by disassembly and storage to air-dry
Hand/skin disinfection with antiseptics	Chemical skin anti- septic 5 ml rubbed for 30–60 seconds (until dry)	Skin cannot be sterilised, only dis- infected with antiseptic Micro-organisms on the skin of patients and caregivers are often associated with infection. Using chemical hand rub is applicable in areas where there is no running water, and in all cases where caregivers look after more than one patient at the same time Antiseptic (waterless) hand rubs can be used before and after touching mucous membranes such as the patient's mouth, non-intact skin or body fluids; or when caring for patients known to be suffering from acute or chronic infections. Use products with sufficient levels of antiseptic or specifically an

Table 8.4 continued

Disinfection process	Contact time/ Holding time	Method
		alcohol-base. Alcohol is less likely to be inactivated in the presence of blood or body fluid than any other antiseptic
		5–10 ml hand disinfectant should be actively rubbed into all the surfaces of the hands, under the fingernails, and left to air-dry
		Active friction is necessary to dislodge organisms from the skin both during skin disinfection and handwashing
		Ingredients for a home made hand rub: 100 ml 70% alcohol with 2 ml glycerine, propylene glycol or sorbitol may be prepared at home and used in small spray/sqeeze bottles that are washed, dried and refilled regularly
		Never use disinfectants or alcohol-based antiseptics (tinctures) on mucous membranes (the genitalia, mouth, ears or eyes) as they are very irritating
		Chlorhexidine gluconate or idiophor (aqueous iodine mixtures) are better choices, but must be used under medical supervision
Disinfecting drinking water	Add 25 ml of clear household bleach to 20 litres of non-municipal water and leave to stand	Use a clean, covered container and filtered water if possible. Polluted water or water which contains large amounts of foreign matter must first

Table 8.4 continued

Disinfection process	Contact time/ Holding time	Method
	for at least one hour Water boiled vigorously (rolling boil) for 5 minutes is generally considered safe to drink. Pour filtered water into a clean clear plastic bottle and wrap a black plastic bag around it. Place in the direct sun for 6 hours (will be pasteurised to ± 65°C and can be used for drinking and baby feeds)	be filtered through a fine cloth and additional bleach (30 ml/20 l water) or chlorine added to reach a 0.1% safety level Using a container with a narrow neck prevents soiled hands or utensils contaminating the water as well as too rapid evaporation of chlorine
Exposure to sunlight	Expose inanimate items as long as possible to sunlight Expose skin to sunlight for no longer than 15 minutes at a time	Sunlight as such does not sterilise, but will dry out surfaces. Most micro-organisms that cause disease won't grow on dry surfaces Airing bedding and mattresses outside and hanging washing in the sun has long been an accepted low level disinfection method Avoid sunburn or exposure of broken skin areas/rashes that will be aggravated by sunlight or heat Wounds and broken skin areas can be exposed to sunlight for a short time, either early in the morning or late in the afternoon when the sun is less strong
Filtration	Immediate effect	Filter liquids such as non-municipal water through special fluid filters, filter paper or finely woven clean

Table 8.4 continued

Disinfection process	Contact time/ Holding time	Method
		cloth/nylon pantyhose This is mostly done before disinfecting or boiling water for washing/ cooking to remove visible foreign material

Food preparation and catering

Nutrition is extremely important in an infection prevention and control programme. Without good nutrition, the patient is unable to produce antibodies, fight off, or cope with infections. Flawless kitchen sanitation, careful food handling, and a high level of personal hygiene are as necessary when caring for a single patient at home as they are when catering for a whole hospital filled with patients.

Immune-suppressed patients are more prone to diarrhoeal infections, while patients with life-limiting diseases often do not have any appetite, cannot face regular meals, or have special dietary requirements such as low protein needs. A terminally ill person may have no appetite, or not need additional nutrition because of a general slowing of all the energy draining life functions, such as digestion. Available finances may also restrict the amount of food and choice of meals. Serving nutritious meals to a patient can become quite a challenge under these circumstances!

Although meals are generally smaller for home-based patients, they may need to be prepared more frequently and stored till needed. Cooking must be done thoroughly – all parts of the food must be heated to the proper temperature, e.g. chicken must be cooked to the bone, without any pink or red meat visible. The holding temperatures of prepared food that is kept should be above 60 °C or below 8 °C, while cooked food that is to be refrigerated must be covered and cooled down as quickly as possible. Cool warm, perishable food before storage or store it in shallow containers to ensure an internal temperature low enough that bacteria will not thrive or produce toxins. Where no refrigerating facilities are available, food should be prepared as needed or stored in a cooler bag, in a cool place under a cloth or wire mesh hood.

Ingredients or dishes served raw, such as salad, must be washed well. Raw fruit and vegetables that can be peeled before serving (bananas, oranges, and cabbage) are better than those that are used whole or just washed. In general, the more immune-suppressed the patient is, the fewer raw ingredients should be used in meals, especially if they have been grown in organic soil fertilized with animal manure. In some cases, processed food such as uncooked meat, biltong, cheese, or yoghurt can cause an infection in a patient with very low resistance.

Supplemental feeds are generally used for patients who cannot eat, or who do not take in enough nourishment, or may need additional nutrients. These feeds can be commercially prepared or home-made. Micro-organisms often contaminate home-made feeds during preparation or during use. Even small numbers of micro-organisms can cause severe diarrhoeal infections. Contaminated equipment, faulty preparation or storage processes, poor technique, or poor hygiene are often to blame.

People who prepare meals or handle food should know:
- the basic principles of personal hygiene and the risk of food-borne disease transmission for each patient they care for
- the importance of reporting their own diarrhoeal diseases or broken skin areas (especially on the hands) to a supervisor to prevent transmission of infections to a patient
- the proper inspection, preparation, and storage procedures of all the food they handle
- how to clean and operate any equipment used
- basic food sanitation and waste management, and
- the basic choice of diet for the specific patient they are caring for.

Education and training

Education is a basic infection control and prevention practice, as caregivers, family members, or outsiders can be exposed to infection because of ignorance or because they have not been taught correctly. Caregivers should make education of the patient and family members a basic element of their routine, starting with basic care giving, and personal or environmental hygiene. Teaching about disease and care is an essential part of care giving, especially where the family is responsible for a portion of the patient's daily care. For example, if the patient has a wound that family members need to dress regularly, they need to know the basic technique(s) as well as the principles of asepsis, such as careful hand washing, working from top to bottom, and from a clean to a contaminated area. This includes infection control measures. Not protecting the family or the patient from infection means that the goal of ensuring the safety of everyone involved with the patient's care has not been achieved, or that risk assessment has not been extensive enough.

Keeping patients (and their families) informed of their progress reassures everyone that there is nothing that cannot be managed in the patient's care and ensures mutual cooperation between patients, caregivers, and family members. Talking is a human function and basic need that should be utilized for the patient's benefit. The caregiver should teach, supervise, revise, and strengthen information and previous knowledge in cooperation with the doctor, other multidisciplinary team members, and the family.

Dying

Remember the saying: 'That which was considered to be infectious during life remains so after death.' After death the patient's blood and body secretions are still considered to be infectious, as well as any drops of blood or body fluid that may leak or be exhaled during the last patient care procedures.

Patients that leak body fluid after death should be wrapped in either linen or plastic sheets, placed in a plastic body bag, or covered well with a waterproof shroud, especially if the fluid is known to be contagious. These bags can be obtained from a funeral home or furniture store.

Disinfection of the environment, the furniture, and the patient care equipment in the place where the patient was cared for until death should be a priority to ensure the safety from infection of everyone left behind. This is the caregiver's final patient care process, as she or he knows what the real infection risk to the remaining family members is. After removal of the patient's remains or when the community comes to view the deceased at home, it is much safer and easier for the family if the environment is already clean and tidy.

Conclusion

Infection control in the home-based care setting is the art of looking after a patient who may be immune-suppressed, living with a life-limiting condition or wounds, or even dying. The process should be based on a standardized programme and set procedures that are applied to each individual in order to assess needs and risks, diagnose problems, and identify and apply solutions, processes, and procedures while teaching and guiding both the patient and the family.

Economic stressors, occupational exposure of health care workers to injuries or infection, and the circumstances of both the patient and caregiver need to be taken into account when standard infection prevention and control measures are chosen to fight suspected or certain infection.

In a written policy that dictates standards of care delivery, the caregiver or service provider should focus on:

- hand washing
- environmental hygiene
- disinfection and sterilization of equipment and surfaces
- preparation of food or catering
- the threat of cross-infection, and
- the possibility or probability of the patient's death.

In all, infection control and prevention becomes a challenge to innovation for both patient and caregiver in the community.

Recommended reading

Association for Professionals in Infection Control and Epidemiology (APIC). 1996. *APIC text of infection control and applied epidemiology – principles and practice.* Washington: APIC.

Association for Professionals in Infection Control and Epidemiology (APIC). 2000. *APIC text of infection control and applied epidemiology – principles and practice.* Washington: APIC.

Cassens, B.J. 1992. *Preventive Medicine and Public Health,* 2nd Edition. Philadelphia: Harwal Publishing.

Pearse, J. 1997. *Infection Control Manual.* Jacana Publishers: Johannesburg.

Ziady, L.E., Small, N., and A.M.J. Louis. 1997. *Infection Control Rapid Reference.* Pretoria: Kagiso Tertiary Publishers.

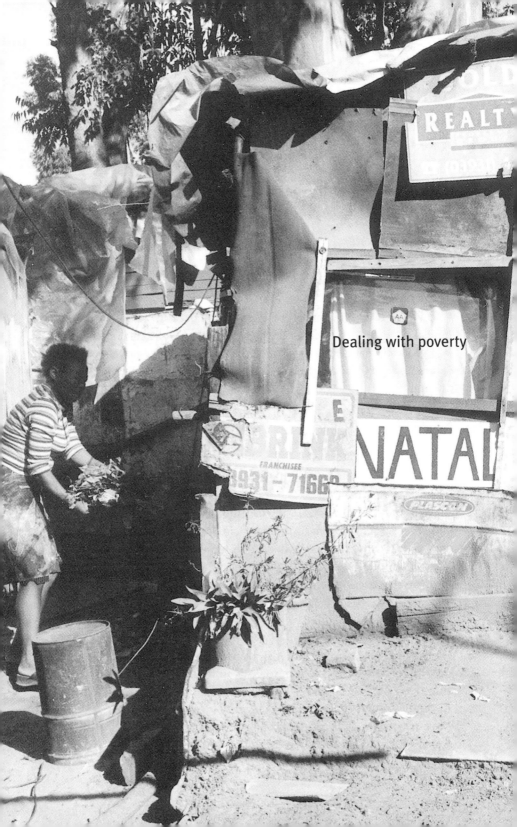

Dealing with poverty

9 | Dealing with poverty

Kath Defilippi

Introduction

The HIV/AIDS pandemic and the associated need for home-based care have forced caregivers to stare into the face of poverty in all its ugliness. This can be a profoundly disturbing experience. In the chapter on global poverty in her book *Reshaping Societies: HIV/AIDS and Social Change*, Susan Hunter comments:

> Income poverty is lack of food, goods, services, opportunities. Moral poverty is lack of physical wellbeing, lack of energy, lack of space, lack of time, lack of power (2000, 123).

There is often also a spiritual dimension to poverty – lack of hope for change or meaning in the midst of suffering.

In a study of home-based care in South Africa, it was found that this is one of the aspects of care that community caregivers (CCGs) found the most difficult to deal with (Uys 2001). Coming into households to assist with care and finding families hungry and cold, without hope of relief, is daunting. If this happens day after day, it may lead to burnout in the CCGs.

Extent of the problem

The link between poverty and AIDS is undisputed. The malnutrition associated with poverty implies a compromised immune status and exposes people to infections such as TB and AIDS. They could, in fact, be described as already having an inherited immunity deficiency syndrome. There is also a lack of basic services, with people sometimes having to walk as far as 4 km to fetch water. This, not surprisingly, results in conditions of poor hygiene that further exacerbate the vulnerability to infection. HIV/AIDS has fuelled TB epidemics in countries where TB was already prevalent. In some developing countries it is estimated that as many as 50 per cent of people may now have TB (Granich and Mermin 1999). The presence of STIs also dramatically increases the risk of transmission of HIV.

Poverty, however, is not just physical. It impacts on social and economic relationships. In parts of sub-Saharan Africa, the unemployment rate is as high as 70 per cent (Defilippi 2000). People feel trapped in a vicious circle of hopelessness. When there is a need to escape the reality of one's dreary existence alcohol and substance abuse, as well as promiscuity, are rife. Domestic violence and sexual abuse are also widespread.

Often, sex is the only means by which a poverty-stricken woman can procure money or food. In sub-Saharan Africa, where gender inequality is culturally entrenched, this is frequently associated with violence and exploitation. It simultaneously advances the spread of HIV. Vulnerability to AIDS is frequently accompanied by a lack of respect for the rights of women and children. Domestic violence increases women's exposure to HIV/AIDS. According to a UNAIDS (2000) report, numerous studies indicate that between a third and a half of married women from many countries and continents are beaten or otherwise physically assaulted by their partners. This leads to a state of subservience that deprives women of the power needed to negotiate safe sex. Women and girls are furthermore frequently denied the right to education and information as well as the right to freedom of expression and association.

A lack of formal education and the resultant low literacy levels combine with the fear and stigma associated with HIV/AIDS to shape the propagation of horrifying myths. The widespread belief that sexual intercourse with a virgin can cure AIDS has led to an increase in the rape of young girls and even infants.

Traditional Zulu culture promotes virginity and expects a married woman to be faithful to her husband. At the same time it is socially acceptable for men to have multiple sexual partners. This apparent contradiction is not restricted to Zulu society. Many societies recommend that women have one sexual partner while men are encouraged to have more (Granich and Mermin 1999). Of the adult AIDS patients referred to South Coast Hospice, 65 per cent are women, 80 per cent of whom have been faithful to their partner according to their own reports. It is probable that these statistics from the southern-most health district of southern KwaZulu-Natal are mirrored in other parts of sub-Saharan Africa.

Almost certainly, the most evil manifestation of poverty is its devastating impact on children. In many parts of sub-Saharan Africa, children's basic rights to food, development, and protection are continually denied by the circumstances of their birth. A child born in a poor family inherits all the ills connected to poverty. They are, more often than not, even deprived of the chance to improve their miserable lot (Hunter 2000). The HIV/AIDS pandemic has greatly intensified the suffering endured by destitute children. Considerable numbers of impoverished children develop HIV/AIDS because of mother-to-child transmission (MTCT). In South Africa it is unusual for these unfortunate children to have access to antiretroviral treatment, and the vast majority will die of an AIDS-related illness at a very young age.

By 2015, almost 12 per cent of the South African population will comprise children who have been orphaned as a result of AIDS. Nearly 61 per cent of all children in the country live in poverty, while 20 per cent do not live with their mothers. According to Hunter,

the chance of being orphaned is three to six times greater than pre-epidemic levels while the likelihood of sexual abuse, exploitation, neglect and malnutrition has increased with the loss of parental protection (2000, 142).

Besides the immediate trauma and risk of contracting HIV, sexual abuse in children holds further implications for spreading the virus. Evidence from high-income countries suggests that sexual abuse of young girls may lead to risky sexual relationships as adolescents. This could be connected to a lowered self-esteem, which would also make it harder for them to be assertive in sexual negotiations in later life.

Family structure is collapsing. More and more children who are themselves traumatized and grieving are heading up orphan households. Invariably these households have to contend with severe poverty with all its horrendous consequences. Elderly women who have worked hard to eke out a living in difficult circumstances are being forced to assume the responsibility of nursing their dying children. The bulk of the burden of care is in fact falling on grandmothers and children – the very segment of society that ought to be receiving protection and care. Scores of grandparents are attempting to stretch their meagre pensions so as to be able to provide food and schooling for their orphaned grandchildren. The quality of parenting that exhausted and impoverished grannies are capable of giving to traumatized children is also often questionable.

Impact on palliative care

The vast majority of PLHA in the developing world do not have access to anti-retroviral therapy. It can, therefore, be implied that they will require and have the right to expect palliative care.

Home-care projects are usually set up to provide home care for bedridden patients. Although poverty impacts directly on the quality of life of patients and their families, organizations should take the following into consideration when deciding what their response to poverty should be:

- *The focus of the organization as portrayed in its mission statement.* It is prudent to maintain focus and keep to the vision encapsulated in the mission statement at all times. It is important to remember that home care itself needs a high level of commitment and input. If the organization tries to be all things to all people, it might fail to accomplish anything. The issue of quality is pivotal for home care to have any long-term meaningful impact on the quality of life of impoverished and seriously ill PLHA and their families.

- *The current skills mix and potential for training and management.* If a project has been built around home care provision, managers and volunteers might not have the required skills to get involved in economic empowerment or poverty alleviation.

- *The availability or potential of other partners in the community to get involved in poverty alleviation.* Networking with other groups and introducing PLHA and families on the home-care programme to groups that can assist with this additional task, is essential. It is important to identify all relevant community resources and establish how best they can be harnessed for the benefit of PLHA, their families, and the entire community. In this way access to a continuum of comprehensive care can be effectively established. In addition to care that extends from pre-diagnosis to bereavement follow-up, PLHA need to have ready access to poverty alleviation and childcare enterprises.

It is suggested that home-based care projects retain their focus on providing quality home-based care, and try to engage other partners to deal with poverty alleviation. Retaining focus and doing one thing really well is beneficial for the recipients of the service as well as to the organization delivering the care. The organization is only able to develop real expertise and credibility if it concentrates on its primary role. The PLHA on the home-care programme benefit by receiving quality care and support for themselves and their families. The home-care team earns the respect of its networking partners. Potential donors are also likely to be impressed by the tangible recognition given to such organizations.

It is not easy to set limits in such a needy environment, particularly when people from the community are providing the hands-on care. Good leadership and management, which ensure good communication to caregivers as well as PLHA, their families and the community, is a prerequisite for success.

Strategies for poverty relief

It is a natural response for caregivers to want to provide hungry people with food. This is only admirable as an emergency measure and is extremely difficult to maintain over the long term. Giving PLHA the power to address the root cause and implement a sustainable solution is definitely preferable.

There is a genuine danger of creating further dependency, and it is important to recognize and avoid this. Criteria for emergency food relief need to be established and adhered to.

Increasing access to social grants

Poor people are also often not aware of their rights and the availability of welfare grants. Across the country, uptake of childcare grants has been identified as a major social welfare problem by the government and other agencies. Currently only a fraction of potential grantees are receiving their grants.

The problems with accessing these grants are numerous, and include:

- obtaining the required documentation, such as identity documents and birth and death certificates
- problems with regard to the availability and cost of transport
- overloaded and unmotivated civil servants and social workers, and
- long queues and poor service in some government departments.

Table 9.1 Grants available in South Africa

Grant name	Monthly payment	Qualification criteria	Documents required	Access procedure
Child support	R140	Child <7 years Parental Income <R1100 (Rural) <R800 (Urban) Maximum of 4 children per carer	Birth certificates ID book of both parents or at least mother Parents' pay slips Immunization cards Letter from Inkosi to ascertain age	Registration at time of birth at home affairs or magistrate's office After birth proof of age needs to be submitted to Dept of Welfare If father not available use mother's surname Apply for grant at social security office
Foster care	R470	Guardian of orphan where both parents have died Child aged 0–18 years Foster parent committed to being legal guardian until child reaches 18 years of age	Death certificates of both parents Marriage certificate of parents Birth certificate of child	Social worker or entrusted associate investigates suitability and writes motivation If father unavailable social worker must handle children's court procedure Quality of care given to child is followed up by social worker or trusted partner NB Grant application can be processed prior to the death of the remaining terminally ill parent

Table 9.1 *continued*

				Grant can be extended to age 21 years if child is dependant e.g. engaged in full-time study
Disability	R640	Adult with significant physical disability e.g. PLHA who is terminally ill	Medical report/ referral letter ID book	Males between 18 and 65 years and females between 18 and 60 years can apply through social security office Grant reviewed regularly to check medical condition Changes to an old age pension
Care dependency	R640	Parent or guardian of child 2–18 years needing continuous care	Medical certificate proving disability of child ID book of mother/guardian Birth certificate of child	District surgeon gives medical certificate Apply for grant at local social security office
Grant in aid	R100	Person already getting old age pension or disability grant who needs intense continuous care e.g. is bedridden	Recipient grant number Social worker's report	Applied for as a bonus to the caregiver Apply at local social security office

Table 9.1 *continued*

Old age pension	R640	Any citizen of pensionable age	ID book	Grant needs to be collected in person,
			Proof of age	and it is available until death
		Males qualify at 65 years, females at 60 years		

Empowering PLHA with information about social grants could have significant impact on the future and potential quality of life for orphans.

Increasing self-reliance with regard to food

An appropriate holistic response would include information about nutrition, food storage and preparation, and motivation about growing fruit and vegetables. PLHA themselves could assist greatly in this area, since they are often not able to work full time, but want to make a contribution and be active.

Community gardens have made a significant contribution to the nutritional status of many families in rural communities all over South Africa. It might be necessary to get assistance for groups to start such gardens, since fencing and getting water to the garden might need some funding. The Department of Agriculture's advice offices are very active in this area and could be contacted in all areas of the country. They might also be able to advise about reputable micro-credit schemes.

Advocacy and lobbying

Every support needs to be given to the community at large and in particular, PLHA groups should be encouraged to become involved in self-help schemes. Credible non-governmental and/or community-based organizations (NGOs/CBOs) are ideally positioned to play an advocacy role in this matter. They can use their influence to persuade political and religious leaders to give such projects their full endorsement.

In addition to becoming politically aware, NGOs and CBOs sometimes need to join PLHA in promoting their human rights. This activist role may also include lobbying for a portion of the formal health care budget to go towards supporting organizations providing home-based care.

Alleviating spiritual poverty

CCGs and professional supervisors involved in giving direct hands-on care are ideally placed to alleviate the suffering associated with spiritual poverty. Care that incorporates genuine respect, acceptance, and compassion helps PLHA and their families to regain a feeling of self worth and dignity. It furthermore often creates an atmosphere that is uniquely open to prayer and the discussion of spiritual burdens such as guilt and shame. Caregivers in the home are frequently the catalyst that results in the PLHA becoming reconciled with his or her church.

The example set by the home-care team may also contribute to lessening the stigma associated with HIV/AIDS. When respectful care is combined with the dissemination of accurate factual information about the spread of HIV, friends and neighbours often become more supportive to PLHA and their families. A feeling of being worthy and a sense of belonging have a profound positive impact on one's spiritual wellbeing.

The encouragement and support given to PLHA regarding the divulgence of their HIV status frequently results in an open and honest family environment that is spiritually liberating. Working with families in the home provides the opportunity for facilitating better communication between members; it also provides an atmosphere that is conducive to encouraging men to take up their responsibility for care (Hunter 2000). When men assume a caring role it may be spiritually beneficial to themselves and can bring joy and gratitude to a dying wife or partner.

Enabling people to deal with unfinished business allows them to die in peace. Children are the primary concern for the vast majority of terminally ill young parents. Mothers in particular find it a great relief when the carer facilitates a discussion about the optimal placement of their children that results in the best possible plan being in place.

Giving culturally sensitive care and support is another potentially powerful tool that CCGs can use to help PLHA and grieving families to attain closure. Once the reality of the situation is honestly confronted it allows emotional energy to be diverted towards maintaining or restoring important relationships. Caregivers can subtly encourage family members in the home to ask for or offer forgiveness to each other. Often the most difficult person to forgive is oneself. This can be facilitated by prayer, tapping into the belief system of the

PLHA, and/or referral to a minister of religion of their choice. A prerequisite of culturally sensitive care is a sincere willingness to avoid trying to impose one's own philosophy of life or religious conviction on the PLHA. It takes a special kind of maturity to be able to support a person in the pursuit of finding meaning in suffering. This need for spiritual maturity and generosity of spirit in caregivers is compounded when the spiritual path of the PLHA and/or family differs from their own.

Linking HIV/AIDS service provision to job creation

The idea of linking HIV/AIDS service provision to job creation needs to be seriously explored in terms of long-term sustainability as well as the impact it is likely to have on reducing poverty in affected communities (Health Development Networks 2001). If poverty alleviation funding comes into communities by paying CCGs, this has a number of advantages:

- It makes an important extension to the formal health service sustainable.
- It creates jobs, not dependency on hand-outs, thus increasing self-respect and self-reliance.
- It facilitates retention of trained CCGs, and thus increases quality of care and lowers costs (of recruitment, selection, training, and orientation).

Conclusion

Reflecting on the magnitude of human suffering, social disruption, and the exacerbation of poverty that the HIV/AIDS pandemic leaves in its wake, it is tempting to link it to the saying 'it is an ill wind that blows no good'. This, however, is not the reality, and it may be helpful to focus on some aspects that impact positively on poverty, be it directly or indirectly. The fact that HIV/AIDS has resulted in the silence surrounding poverty to be broken is an essential first step in the process of addressing this seemingly overwhelming problem.

References

Defilippi, K.M. 2000. 'Palliative care issues in sub-Saharan Africa'. *International Journal of Palliative Nursing* 6 (3): 108.

Granich, R. and J. Mermin. 1999. *HIV Health and Your Community*. Stanford: Stanford University Press.

Health Development Networks. 2001. 'Findings and Recommendations', proceedings of the first *Southern African Regional Community Home Based Care Conference.* Gabarone: Botswana Government Printers.

Hunter, S.S. 2000. *Reshaping Societies: HIV/AIDS and Social Change.* New York: Hudson Run Press.

UNAIDS. 2000. *Report on the Global HIV/AIDS Epidemic.* Geneva: UNAIDS.

Uys, L.R. 2001. 'The implementation of the integrated community-based home care model for people living with AIDS'. *African Journal of Nursing and Midwifery* 3 (1): 34–41.

Recommended reading

Campbell, L. 2001. *Interim Report on HIV/AIDS/STD/TB Pilot Site in UGU South Health District.* Port Shepstone: South Coast Hospice.

Gie, R., Schaaf, H., and J. Barnes. 1993. 'The socio-economic determinants of the AIDS epidemic in South Africa: A cycle of poverty'. *South African Medical Journal* 83: 223–4.

Mnguni, M.B. 2002. *Impact of HIV/AIDS on Infected and Affected Women in Rural Areas.* Unpublished assignment for Hospice Association of South Africa short course in palliative nursing care. Port Shepstone: South Coast Hospice.

Mzolo, B.K.2002. 'Sympathetic soul'. *Nursing Update* 25 (12): 18–19.

Van der Walt, H. 2000. 'STH Consortium (Sungardens, Tateni, Hospivision) Community Empowerment Project'. Proceedings of the Bristol-Meyers Squibb Home-based Care Conference, Pretoria, November.

Planning for orphans
and HIV/AIDS affected
children

Planning for orphans and HIV/AIDS affected children

10

Rose Smart

Introduction

Definitions abound for orphans, affected children, children in distress (CINDI), children affected by AIDS (CABA), and orphans and vulnerable children (OVC). The following terms are used in this chapter. However, these terms are subject to ongoing debate.

Orphan: a child under the age of fifteen who has lost his or her mother. (Orphans are sometimes described as maternal, paternal, or double orphans.)

An infected child: a child who is infected with HIV (vertically – which means from mother to child – sexually, or from unsafe health practices).

An affected child: a child living in a household in which there are, or have been, one or more HIV-infected family members.

Global facts

In 2001, UNAIDS released the following facts regarding children and HIV/AIDS:

- HIV/AIDS has orphaned at least 13 million children currently under fifteen years of age. The total number of children orphaned by the pandemic since it began is forecast to almost double to 25 million by 2010.
- AIDS-related deaths caused some 2.3 million children to become orphans in 2000 (one every fourteen seconds!). UNICEF estimates that up to a third of these children were less than five years old.
- An estimated 10.3 million people aged fifteen to twenty-four are living with HIV/AIDS, and half of all new infections – over 7 000 daily – are occurring among young people.

- In some of the worst-affected countries, adolescent girls are being infected at a rate five to six times higher than are boys.

The situation in sub-Saharan Africa

HIV/AIDS is eroding precious and hard-won infant and child survival gains. In the world's nine most severely-affected countries (all of them located in Africa), where at least one-tenth of the adult population has HIV, life expectancy for a child born in 2000–2005 will drop to forty-three years from the pre-AIDS expectancy of sixty years of life. The United States Bureau of the Census estimates that by the year 2010, HIV/AIDS may increase the infant mortality rate (IMR) by 76 per cent and the under-five mortality rate (U5MR) by more than 100 per cent in those regions most affected.

In most parts of the industrialized world usually no more than 1 per cent of the child population is orphaned. Before the onset of HIV/AIDS, societies in the developing world absorbed orphans into extended families and communities at a rate of just over 2 per cent of the child population (between 2 and 5 per cent in South Africa), and traditionally orphanhood was not perceived to be a problem. Today, because of HIV/AIDS, the situation is vastly different.

Table 10.1 Orphans as a percentage of children under fifteen in 2000

Country	%	Country	%
Botswana	15.1%	Lesotho	17.0%
Malawi	17.5%	South Africa	10.3%
Zambia	17.6%	Zimbabwe	17.6%

Source: UNAIDS, UNICEF and USAID (2002)

Sub-Saharan Africa is currently confronting the reality of:

- increasing numbers of orphans and affected children associated with the escalating HIV/AIDS pandemic
- the inability of traditional models of surrogate child care to accommodate the number of orphaned and affected children, and
- the inability of poor communities to absorb orphans into informal care facilities without the introduction of outside support.

The impact of HIV/AIDS on families and communities

For generations, the extended family system has met most of the basic needs of children and provided a protective social environment in which they could grow and develop. Kinship systems have dictated various social, economic, and religious obligations towards the family lineage as well as the social and material rights of the individual within the lineage.

Social upheaval, rapid urbanization, war, drought, famine, and acute political and economic stress have threatened the integrity of the extended family and have undermined its efficacy as a social support network. For the extended family, additional children increase financial hardships and pressures on relationships, weakening the capacity of the family to cope. The overriding constraint to the care of additional children, therefore, is the capacity of the extended family to cope.

At a time when the family is most needed as a support system for orphans and affected children, the stigma associated with HIV/AIDS is further affecting the willingness of families to care for and support these children. This is resulting in increased child mobility and the exploitation and neglect of children.

The impact of the pandemic on children

Neither words nor statistics can adequately capture the human tragedy of children grieving for dying or dead parents stigmatised by society through association with HIV/AIDS, plunged into economic crisis and insecurity by their parents' death, and struggling without services or support systems in impoverished communities (UNICEF 1999, 8).

Orphans and affected children are even more vulnerable than adults, as they face the possibility of stigma relating to their own status, if they are infected, as well as stigma flowing from their parent's or caregiver's status. This stigma often continues even after the death of their caregiver, when they are rejected or treated with scorn by the extended family and the community.

Research has also shown that stigma and discrimination lead to orphans and affected children being denied or discouraged from accessing basic services, such as health care and welfare services.

The reality of HIV/AIDS in the family is that children are caring for the sick and assuming adult responsibilities before they are ready to do so. Children are leaving school earlier, they marry earlier, enter the labour force earlier, and are frequently sexually exploited.

The term 'parentification' refers to the process of creating a parent out of a child in order to care for a parent or siblings. This is associated with social isolation. Younger children not only assume responsibility for more complex household chores, but are also deprived of the nurturing previously received from their now ill parents.

When my mother is sick we become sad with my sister. I think I am afraid. We cry sometimes. I am afraid my grandmother is also sick – Boy whose mother is living with HIV/AIDS (Clacherty & Associates 2001, 41).

- HIV/AIDS produces younger orphans and these younger children are especially at risk.
- They tend to be nutritionally deprived (at a time when they have higher nutritional needs).
- In many communities, children whose parents have died of AIDS are at greater risk of dying of preventable diseases, because their illnesses tend to be attributed to AIDS and thus go untreated.
- Orphans are also less likely than other children to be immunized and to have their health care needs adequately met.

Unless suitable arrangements are made for children before their parents' deaths, the trauma, guilt, and grief so common among these children is compounded by uncertainty regarding their future.

When the extended family either does not exist or simply cannot cope, the only alternative is often for siblings to live together, frequently with no adult supervision. Child-headed households have their own unique problems, which include:

- poverty
- lack of supervision and care
- stunting and hunger
- educational failure
- lack of adequate medical care
- psychological problems
- disruption of normal childhood and adolescence
- exploitation
- early marriage
- discrimination
- poor housing, and
- child labour.

Framework for developing a response to orphans and affected children

There is now global consensus that children's rights need special protection. The aim is to focus on the whole child and promote the effective realization of all his or her rights. This is the framework for working with children affected by HIV/AIDS, augmented by an understanding of the needs of the orphans, their guardians, and the communities in which they live.

The rights of children

In 1989, a decade after the International Year of the Child, the United Nations General Assembly adopted the Convention on the Rights of the Child (CRC), which sets out the political, civil, cultural, economic, and social rights of children. A decade later all the countries of the world except two (USA and Somalia) have ratified it. The CRC guarantees the rights of children to:

- protection (from maltreatment, neglect, and all forms of exploitation)
- provision (of food, health care, education, social security), and
- participation (in all matters concerning them).

These in turn have defined the four principles of the CRC:
- non-discrimination
- the best interests of the child
- the right to life, survival, and development, and
- respect for the views of the child.

Among the rights defined in the CRC are many that have particular relevance in the context of HIV/AIDS.

Children's rights with HIV/AIDS implications

Survival and development
An inherent right to life and efforts to ensure a child's survival and development.

Separation from parents
The right to live with their parents, unless this is incompatible with their best interests.

The child's opinion and freedom of expression
A child has a right to express an opinion, and to have that opinion considered, in any matter or procedure affecting the child.
A child has a right to obtain and make known information, and to express his or her views, unless this would violate the rights of others.

Protection of privacy
Children should be protected from interference with their privacy regarding their families, homes, and correspondence.

Access to appropriate information
The media has a responsibility to disseminate information to children that is consistent with their moral wellbeing, that fosters knowledge and understanding between people, and that respects children's cultural backgrounds.

Protection from abuse and neglect
Protect children from all forms of maltreatment perpetuated by parents and others responsible for their care.

Protection of children without families and adoption
Provide special protection for children deprived of their family environment and ensure that appropriate, alternative family care or institutional placement is made available to them, taking into account the child's cultural background.
Adoption shall only be carried out in the best interests of the child.

Children with disabilities
Children with disabilities have a right to special care, education, and training designed to help them achieve the greatest possible self-reliance and lead full active lives in society.

Health and health services
Children have a right to the highest level of health possible, which includes the right to health and medical services, with special emphasis on pri-

mary and preventive health care, public health education, and the diminution of infant mortality.

Social security and standard of living

Children have a right to benefit from social security.

Children have a right to benefit from an adequate standard of living.

Education, leisure, recreation, and cultural activities

A child has a right to education – ensure that at least primary education is free and compulsory.

Children have a right to leisure and play and to participate in cultural and artistic activities.

Child labour

Protect children from engaging in work that constitutes a threat to their health, education, or development.

Sexual exploitation and drug abuse

Children have a right to protection from sexual exploitation and abuse, including prostitution and involvement in pornography.

Children have a right to protection from narcotic and psychotropic drugs and from being involved in their production or distribution.

Torture and deprivation of liberty, and armed conflict

Children should be treated appropriately, separated from detained adults, allowed contact with family, and given access to legal and other assistance.

No child under fifteen should take a direct part in hostilities or be recruited into the armed forces.

Source: Adapted from Skelton 1998

The needs of orphans, guardians, and communities

All children have physical, emotional, social, and intellectual needs that must be met if they are to enjoy life, develop their full potential, and develop into participating, contributing adults. If any one of these basic needs remains unmet – or is inadequately met – then development may become stunted or distorted.

The needs of orphans are multiple, extending far beyond physical and material needs. Typically their needs include the need for food and security, housing, clothing and bedding, health care, education and income generation, parenting, friends and recreation, and non-discrimination and legal protection.

Guardians also may have wide-ranging needs. Not only may they need assistance with physical work, they may also have many material needs. In addition, these guardians will need counselling, education, and social support.

The need for 're-training' in parenting skills of grandmothers caring for orphaned or affected children, is often overlooked.

And finally, the community itself needs help in coping. Caregivers should help to establish systems to identify and monitor orphans and affected children and needy families and to supervise the care of children.

Supporting organizations such as the church or women's organizations may involve administrative and technical assistance and training, or help in coordinating non-governmental organizations (NGOs) involved in programmes caring for these children.

Models of care and support

Community involvement

There is general consensus that interventions to assist orphans and affected children should be based in, and owned by, the affected communities themselves.

- Members of the community are in the best position to know which households are most severely affected and what sort of help is appropriate. They know who is dying, who has died, who has been taken in by relatives, who is living alone, and who has enough to eat.
- Volunteers from within the community are more likely to visit households regularly and the help they offer is more likely to be practical and supportive. The role of outside organizations is to assist communities by capacity building.

Classification of models

Models of care and support for orphans and affected children can be classified. During the review of the Child Care Act, the South African Law Commission described the different models as follows:

- independent living by orphans
- independent living with external supervision and support

- foster care including traditional family care, cluster care of multiple children, and collective care of individuals or multiple children
- adoption
- institutional care including places of safety, shelters, short-term infant homes, and traditional children's homes, and
- state- or NGO-sponsored community-based support structures including feeding posts and day-care facilities.

Family and community-based approaches appear to best meet the child's need for security and socialization, however they need to be supported and strengthened if they are to remain a viable way of meeting all the needs of the child.

In order for informal caregivers to be able to meet the basic survival needs of children in their care they need access, at the very least, to functioning health, education, and social services.

Orphanages are not generally the most appropriate intervention for orphans and affected children as they can fail to meet children's developmental and emotional needs. While orphanages may be the only option for some children, in general it is better to devote resources towards strengthening the abilities of families and communities to care for orphaned and affected children.

Minimum standards

Although the concept of minimum standards is often contentious, it is useful to consider possible minimum standards of care and support for orphans and affected children. The following were developed as part of a South African study commissioned by UNICEF in 2000 (Loening-Voysey and Wilson 2000).

Essential elements

Food

Nutritious and balanced diet with three meals a day as an absolute minimum

Involving children in the preparation and choice of food (which creates opportunities for participation and for teaching the child important life skills)

Clothing

At least one change of clothing that offers protection against the elements

Nappies for infants

Home environment

Shelter against the elements and protection against environmental and other hazards

A personal and safe sleeping space that provides privacy for older children and protection for all children

Basic household amenities and cleanliness

Spare bedding

Education/schooling

Schooling from age seven to fifteen years, even where there are no funds for school fees or a school uniform

Time to go to school and time and space to do homework

An adult caregiver or older child available to do homework with the child

Entrepreneurship skills training for older children to increase their capacity for self-sufficiency

Hygiene/infection control

Facilities for personal hygiene practices

Universal precaution materials and guidance where there is a risk of infection

Access to water and sanitation

Treatment and health care

Immunization and recording in the Road to Health card

Access to basic treatment and health care

Reliable caregiver to administer medicines, dietary supplements, and home remedies as directed

Reliable caregiver who is aware of, and can respond to, indications of illness and needs for basic first aid

Protection

Against discrimination, stigmatization, abuse, and neglect

Arrangements for the care of the child before the parent dies, including drawing up a will, nominating a legal guardian for the child, and stipulating the child's inheritance

A caring, constant, and reliable adult presence to whom the child can disclose abuse, and who can access help for the child

Healthy discipline practices including setting rules and limits

Affection

A caring, constant, and reliable adult presence who offers security and continuity and with whom the child can communicate openly

An adult caregiver with a positive communication style, which includes 'being there' for the child, taking time to listen and communicate at the child's level

Identity
Birth registration
Retaining and respecting the child's name, kinship, and identity
Capturing memories for the child such as photos, artefacts, details of significant others, and cultural connections
Acknowledging the individuality of the child, for example celebration of birthdays
Participation
Adult caregivers who discuss care plans with the child and get their contribution to these plans
Opportunities for children to participate in all decisions affecting their lives
Decision-making that involves the child around their care plan and that provides a sense of security and protection as well as a sense of future
Understanding, information and communication
Training for children in basic survival skills and life skills
Caregivers who are able to communicate, at least on a basic level, with children in the language of their community of origin (to foster a sense of belonging, cultural connection, and identity for the child)
Information and open communication with children about their own health status if HIV-positive
Information and open communication with children on health issues, including sexuality and relationships
Counselling/supportive services
Support and guidance for children who are experiencing social and emotional difficulties. Where caregivers are unable to do this, access to appropriate assistance
Open communication with children about death, of a parent, family member, friend, or their own death, and emotional and spiritual support
After-death services, including transport of body to mortuary and a dignified burial
Recreation/leisure
Balance between household chores, recreation, and leisure time
Time to play and be able to be children
Freedom of expression
The time and opportunities to question and discuss values, ethics, and morals and to be able to freely seek information and express their ideas

Guidelines

Guidelines from actual programmes offer useful examples, which can be adapted and used in other contexts. The guidelines selected cover:
- mechanisms for identifying and assessing orphans and affected children and defining roles and responsibilities
- principles of, and strategies for, community-based care and support programmes for orphans and affected children
- training and capacity building needs of orphans and affected children, and
- indicators and methods of monitoring and evaluating programmes of care and support for orphans and affected children.

Mechanisms for identifying and assessing orphans and affected children and defining roles and responsibilities

Research commissioned by Bambisanani (Mabude 2000), a rural HIV/AIDS programme in South Africa, made the following recommendations related to a proposed model for identifying orphans and affected children:
- Collaboration as well as role definition for each identified organization in the model is critical.
- Community child care committees (CCCCs) should be established in all administrative areas, to ensure that orphans, affected children, and their families are identified early and offered the necessary support.
- A standardized form should be developed for use in the identification of orphans and affected children.
- A register of orphans and affected children should be established and maintained.
- Care supporters (involved in home-based care) should be given further training so as to be effective in their diverse roles, including those related to identifying and supporting orphans and affected children.
- The need to appoint district CINDI coordinators was stressed.
- Orphans and affected children should receive support such as meals, homework supervision, training to care for ill parents, counselling, peer group activities, life skills training, and income-generating skills at the drop-in centres.

A base-line assessment of orphans and affected children can include:
- How are orphans and affected children perceived by the community?
- Who talks/listens to children? Who do children talk/listen to?

- Are the numbers and/or needs of orphans and affected children increasing?
- How do households with orphans and affected children cope?
- Who do they call on for assistance?

Practical criteria that can be used to identify the children in greatest need can be identified by community members. The following list is an example of such criteria:

- children living on their own with no adult supervision/guidance
- children living with a terminally ill parent
- children looked after by an elderly grandparent
- children dirty or in rags
- children with a withdrawn appearance
- hut in poor state of repair
- lack of chickens or other animals; no crops
- no food in the hut and no sign of recent fire for cooking, and
- children not attending school.

In 1996, community workshops were held in Zambia as part of a UNICEF-funded process to identify innovative or indigenous models of care for orphaned and affected children (McKerrow 1996). A four-tier response was identified, which is useful for clarifying roles and responsibilities at different levels:

- The family must identify affected children and orphans and provide the basic day-to-day needs of the children as well as emotional support.
- The community must support both the children and their caretakers as well as act as a forum for lobbying authorities to assist in providing an effective response.
- Churches, NGOs and community-based organizations (CBOs) must coordinate all responses while also providing material support and support services.
- The state must develop local infrastructure; empower state personnel; create an enabling environment at all levels; modify state services; and facilitate funding for grass-roots services.

Principles and strategies for community-based programmes for orphans and affected children

The following principles were identified and adopted to guide responses to orphans and affected children in Zambia.

- Orphans must not be targeted in isolation from other vulnerable children. Stigma and discrimination associated with HIV/AIDS are lessened when a project is not AIDS-specific.
- Siblings should remain together.
- Children should, as far as possible, remain in their homes or communities of origin.
- Caretakers must be supported through skills training in income-generating activities and child care skills.
- Development of communities is invariably a greater priority for communities, and programmes focusing on vulnerable children must ideally be linked to development programmes.
- Communities must provide support systems for both children and their caretakers.
- Criteria must be developed at community level for identifying the recipients of aid.
- NGOs should work through local CBOs.
- In the delivery of child-centred programmes, links to other service or care programmes catering for the sick, the elderly, the handicapped, etc. are invaluable.
- Use must be made of locally recruited coordinators and volunteers who must receive appropriate training and supervision.
- Responses must facilitate the provision of both direct and indirect aid packages.
- Support that benefits the entire community is preferable.
- State resources must be made user-friendly.
- Simplifying procedures, such as fostering and adoption procedures and access to grants will greatly enhance support for orphans and affected children.

There are a number of key strategies that are required for a community-based response to orphans and affected children to succeed. These include:
- Raising awareness about the problem.
- Documenting the extent of the problem by:
  - assessing the needs
  - keeping a register of orphans
  - finding out what communities can do themselves, and
  - checking on progress.
- Mobilizing the community for action by:

- identifying who in the community is already involved in responding to the needs of the OVC
- identifying who has the interest or capacity to be more involved
- developing partnerships with outside organizations
- networking, and
- mobilizing volunteers from the affected community.
- Making ends meet by:
  - saving labour
  - directly increasing household income
  - relieving the burden (with cash grants, food aid, school fees, agricultural inputs, blankets, and other essential items), and
  - indirect measures (such as protecting the property and inheritance rights of women and children).
- Helping to educate and train children.
- Improving legal systems to help children by:
  - protecting children from exploitation, and
  - making it easier to get help.

Some form of support is always required, and it is necessary to identify what support is needed and who needs it by using a checklist such as the following:
Support parents with:

- practical, emotional, and material assistance
- day care and relief care for children
- health care for children
- education and stimulation for children
- making a will to protect children, and
- selecting a guardian.

Support child-headed households by:

- providing practical, nutritional, health, financial and/or material assistance
- providing developmental, emotional, spiritual, and social support
- ensuring that educational, training, and recreational needs are met, and
- facilitating guardianship arrangements.

Support the extended family with:

- training, counselling, and supervision (if necessary)
- assistance in obtaining resources

- assistance with income generation (if necessary), and
- facilitating guardianship arrangements.

Promote informal foster care for children without families by:
- mobilizing foster carers in communities
- obtaining community agreement for volunteers to foster children
- training, support, and supervision for caregivers
- helping to obtain the necessary resources, and
- facilitating guardianship arrangements.

Training and capacity building for orphans and affected children

Every programme of care and support for orphans and affected children should include training to enable the children to cope more effectively with the situation in which they find themselves or to undertake the roles they are required to fulfil.

The Salvation Army in Zimbabwe runs three types of training camps for orphans (Parry 1998):
- life skills and coping capacity camps with the aim of rebuilding their confidence and helping them to overcome the loss of their parents
- teenage parenting courses to equip orphans looking after their siblings with positive parenting skills, knowledge of children's rights, hygiene, nutrition and first aid, and
- vocational training programmes in arts, crafts and hospitality, and catering management.

An extensive study into the education system in Swaziland made a number of recommendations related to securing the rights of orphans and affected children to education (King 1999):
- Offer exemptions to homesteads/institutions with orphans and affected children to enable children to attend school; waiving school uniform requirements when affordability is a problem; expanding school-based feeding programmes for schoolchildren; and introducing flexible schooling hours, where possible, to keep children in school who might otherwise have to drop out because of labour requirements elsewhere.
- Increase day-care facilities, particularly at the schools, to allow class attendance by children who would otherwise have to take care of their younger siblings.

- Create an educational insurance scheme permitting parents to invest in policies catering for their children's school fees in the event of their death.
- Use national funds as an investment in the education of children.

Monitoring and evaluating programmes of care and support for orphans and affected children

It is important to encourage regular critical analysis of needs/actions and to integrate monitoring and evaluation into routine programme operations. Some possible methodologies and sources of data for such exercises are as follows:

- Simple participatory systems can be used to provide useful data for both community organizations and for donor reporting.
- Volunteers can maintain valuable records of activities.
- Regular group feedback can be useful for peer support, motivation and peer review of decisions/actions.
- Supervisory visits can serve to confirm activities/support and to identify instances where support is insufficient or absent.

Conclusion

There are challenges to successful care and support for orphans and vulnerable children that need to be highlighted. Community mobilization is more challenging in urban areas than in rural areas. Children are often not seen by communities as an important stakeholder group. This is particularly evident in the exclusion of children when there is a death in the family. Orphans and affected children, especially young females, are extremely vulnerable to sexual abuse and exploitation.

Many key lessons about the care of orphans have been learnt over the past decade. These should be heeded if we want to secure the future of the next generation.

References

Clacherty & Associates. 2001. *The Role of Stigma and Discrimination in Increasing the Vulnerability of Children and Youth Infected with and Affected by HIV/AIDS*. Report on a series of workshops. Arcadia, UK: Save the Children.

King, J.T. 1999. *Impact Assessment of HIV/AIDS on the Education Sector.* Report commissioned by the Ministry of Education, Swaziland.

Loening-Voysey, H. and T. Wilson. 2000. *Approaches to Caring for HIV/AIDS Orphans and Vulnerable Children: Essential Elements for a Quality Service.* Unpublished report. Geneva: UNICEF.

Mabude, Z. 2000. *Bambisanani – Identification of Children in Distress.* Kokstad: Bambisanani Project.

McKerrow, N. 1996. *Implementation Strategies for the Development of Models of Care for Orphaned Children.* Unpublished consultation report, commissioned by UNICEF, Zambia.

Parry, S. 1998. *Farm Orphans: Who is Coping?* Zimbabwe: FOST.

Skelton, A (ed.). 1998. *Children and the Law.* Pretoria: Lawyers for Human Rights.

UNAIDS, UNICEF and USAID. 2002. *Children on the Brink.* Geneva: UNAIDS.

UNICEF. 1999. *Children Orphaned by AIDS: Front-line Responses from Eastern and Southern Africa.* Geneva: UNICEF.

Recommended reading

UNAIDS. 2001. *Children and Young People in a World of AIDS.* Geneva: UNAIDS.

Appendices

Appendix A: Media policy of South Coast Hospice

In terms of the South Coast Hospice Procedures Manual, it is a requirement that this policy be read and agreed to by all journalists, reporters, photographers, broadcasters, and film makers visiting patients and families in the care of South Coast Hospice, or when interviewing any volunteers or members of staff.

As a registered non-profit organization, South Coast Hospice welcomes the scrutiny of the media in terms of how funds are deployed. We also appreciate that publicity can lead to additional resources for the enhancement and sustainability of our care programmes.

At the same time we acknowledge the sanctity of our relationship of trust with patients and families and strive to maintain confidentiality at all times. South Coast Hospice (SCH) can therefore only be used as a means of establishing contact with individual patients and families when:

- It is accepted that patients and family members who give consent prior to any interview are free to withdraw such consent at any time. Should this occur, the relevant member of the media may need to wait in a vehicle whilst the patient is tended by SCH staff or volunteers.
- There is total clarity with regard to what, where, when and how the interview will be published or broadcast.
- Names and photographs may only be used after the full implications are made clear to the patient and family by the SCH professional who accompanies the media representative.
- Patients, particularly minors, must always be afforded the opportunity of consulting with family and/or community leaders if they so wish, prior to

consenting to either an interview or photography.

- Any follow-up visits to patients and families are arranged through the Executive Director or the relevant Head of Department (HOD).

South Coast Hospice makes extensive use of trained community members in the delivery of hands-on care, counselling and support. Prior to granting a media interview all staff members and volunteers require written authorization from the CEO, Deputy Director or relevant HOD.

We welcome the opportunity of checking the accuracy of clinical or organizational information prior to publication of the text.

As a general rule visits need to be arranged at least two weeks in advance.

Source: South Coast Hospice, Port Shepstone

Appendix B: Job description for a community caregiver at South Coast Hospice

Job description:	Hospice caregiver (HIV/AIDS project)
Appointment:	Project supervisor after consultation with care coordinator
Mission:	To provide high-quality holistic and professional care to the patients and families referred to South Cost Hospice AIDS Home-care project
Key performance areas:	
1 Clinical	Providing good basic nursing care to patients as directed by a project supervisor, including unscheduled after-hours care when on call
	Using communication skills to facilitate openness and honesty
2 Administration	Attending meetings and keeping records and statistics as prescribed by project supervisors/care coordinator
3 Promotion	To actively promote a positive public image for South Coast Hospice and the project
4 Education	Teach and empower families and the community to care for patients as well as themselves Actively promote the acceptance of AIDS as an illness without stigma
Qualifications:	Basic hospice training including practical
Organizational relationships:	Upwards: • project supervision • hospice home care sister • care coordinator • hospice administrator Horizontal: • other caregivers on team

Functional liaison:	Patient and family Community Fellow caregivers on the team Project supervisors
Authority:	To use own initiative to alert project supervisor to any problem Suggest contact with a minister of religion Facilitate community support Implement prescribed treatment regimes Borrow hospice equipment
Limitation of authority:	May not accept referrals to the project without consulting project supervisor May not arrange admission of patient without consulting project supervisor May not give formal talks without consulting project supervisor May not acquire or dispose of assets of South Coast Hospice
Performance standards:	
Clinical key performance area:	Well catered-for patient who is comfortable and able to communicate with his/her family Family coping and pulling together Appropriate and competent use of hospice vehicle and equipment
Administration key performance area:	Clear record of visits Transport forms accurately completed
Promotion key performance area:	Community acceptance of project Professional approach and strict adherence to confidentiality resulting in maintenance of hospice's good reputation in the community

Project supervisor: .... **Care coordinator:** ....

Date: .... **Date:** ....

Appendix C: First assessment form for patients at South Coast Hospice's community-based home-care programme

Assessment

Patient assessment:	Date:
Surname:	Date of birth:
First name:	ID no:
Likes to be known as:	
What religion were you brought up in:	
Current religion:	Minister:
Address:	
Tel no:	Ethnic origin:
Next of kin:	Address:
Surname:	Tel. No (h):

First name:	Tel no (w):
Address	
Primary caregiver:	Age:
Relationship to patient:	
Hospital:	Current medicine:
OPD number:	Clinic:
CBOs involved:	
Organization:	
Allergies:	
Referred by hospital clinic:	

Contact person:	Tel no:
Other hospice team involved:	

Presenting symptoms

Thrush	Pneumonia	TB
Dysphagia	Vomiting	Wounds
Skin rashes	Nausea	Diarrhoea
Sweating	Drowsiness	
Weight loss	Confusion	Malignancy
Coughing	Mental status	
Dry mouth	Dyspnoea	
Weakness	Anorexia	
Sleeping		

What health education was given?
Is the family aware of client's status?
When:
Relationship to client:
Mobililty:

General comments:

Assessor's name: Date:

Genogram

ME of child	Age	Gender	Going to school Yes/no	Birth cert/ID Yes/no	Involved in caregiving	Relation-ship to patient	Time for play Yes/No	Will this child be an orphan?
1								
2								
3								
4								
5								
6								
7								
8								
9								
10								

Plans made for children after death of patient

Index